INSTRUCTOR'S RESOURCE MANUAL FOR

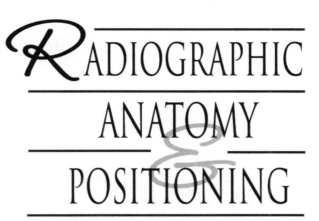

RADIOGRAPHIC ANATOMY & POSITIONING

An Integrated Approach

Mary L. Madigan, RT (R) (M)
Clinical Coordinator
Radiologic Technology Program
Bellevue Community College
Bellevue, Washington

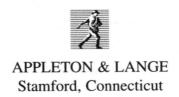

APPLETON & LANGE
Stamford, Connecticut

Copyright © 1998 by Appleton & Lange
A Simon & Schuster Company

98 99 00 01 02/ 10 9 8 7 6 5 4 3 2 1

Prentice Hall International (UK) Limited, *London*
Prentice Hall of Australia Pty. Limited, *Sydney*
Prentice Hall Canada, Inc., *Toronto*
Prentice Hall Hispanoamericana, S.A., *Mexico*
Prentice Hall of India Private Limited, *New Delhi*
Prentice Hall of Japan, Inc., *Tokyo*
Simon & Schuster Asia Pte, Ltd., *Singapore*
Editora Prentice Hall do Brasil Ltda., *Rio de Janeiro*
Prentice Hall, *Upper Saddle River, New Jersey.*

ISBN: 0–8385–8245–1

Acquisitions Editor: Kim Davies
Production Editor: Elizabeth Ryan
Designer: Janice Barsevich Bielawa

PRINTED IN THE UNITED STATES OF AMERICA

ISBN: 0-8385-8245-1
90000

9 780838 582459

CONTENTS

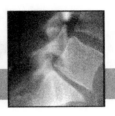

INTRODUCTION

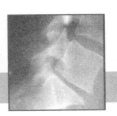

This *Instructor's Resource Manual* accompanies the textbook *Radiographic Anatomy & Positioning: An Integrated Approach* by Andrea Gauthier Cornuelle and Diane H. Gronefeld, and the *Applications Manual* by Diane H. Gronefeld and Mary L. Madigan. The purpose of the *Instructor's Resource Manual* is to help ease the transition for experienced instructors from a familiar textbook to a new, unfamiliar one. It also should prove to be a valuable resource for instructors teaching this course for the first time.

The book is divided into three sections, and each chapter is organized in the following way:
Objectives
Chapter Outline
Sample 50-Minute Lesson
    Preparation
    Presentation
    Application
    Testing
Exam Questions
Answer Key
Answer Key/Solutions for the *Applications Manual*

The first section of the *Instructor's Resource Manual* contains a page comparison of the textbook with other commonly used texts. There is also a quarter system sample course outline and a semester system sample course outline. As you can see by looking at the outlines, the text can be presented in a rapid manner, as in the quarter system outline, or at a more relaxed pace, as in the semester system outline. How the text is presented would depend on the time allotted in the curriculum for this material and the aptitude of the particular class. The text works very well for both methods of presentation. Although both outlines follow the chapters in sequence, they could be taught in any order that would best serve a particular program.

The second section includes material from the eighteen chapters in *Radiographic Anatomy & Positioning: An Integrated Approach,* and the answers to the study questions and puzzles contained in the *Applications Manual.* The *Instructor's Resource Manual* also contains a discussion about the case studies presented in the *Applications Manual.* Moreover, there is a detailed list of objectives and a sample 50-minute teaching outline for each chapter.

The third section contains transparency masters from the text which would be useful in the presentation of this material.

This *Instructor's Resource Manual* has been carefully crafted to provide you with the tools to build a system of customized instruction. Appleton & Lange realizes that there are many radiographic anatomy and positioning books on the market from which to choose. Our goal is to help you make your textbook changes as easy as possible. Your feedback while using this guide is much appreciated.

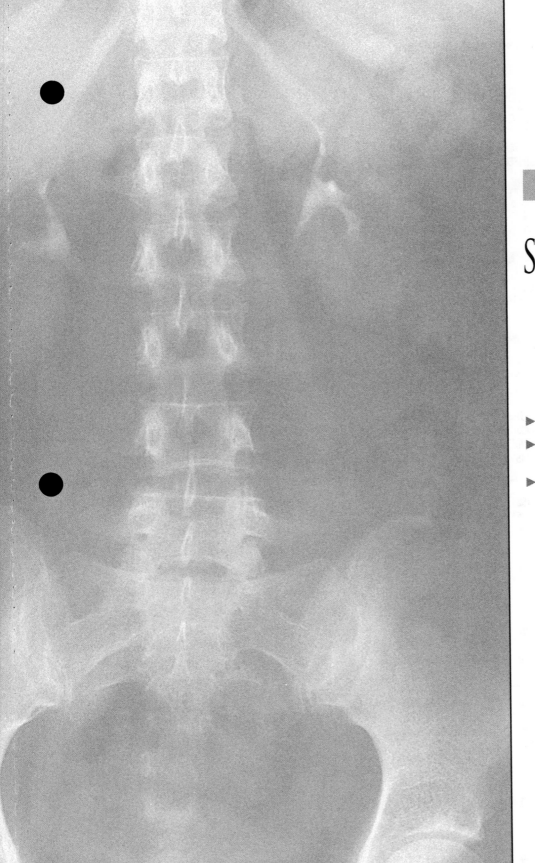

1

SECTION

► PAGE COMPARISON OF TEXTBOOK BY CORNUELLE & GRONEFELD WITH OTHER COMMONLY USED TEXTS

	CORNUELLE & GRONEFELD	BALLINGER	BONTRAGER	EISENBERG
Chest		**Volume 1**		
Anatomy	30–34	436–441	55–63	23–25
Procedural Considerations	34–43	442–445	65–71	—
Projections	45–53	476–479	72–84	26–35
Abdomen		**Volume 2**		
Anatomy	58–68	32–35	85–91	213–216
Procedural Considerations	68–73	36–37	92–93	—
Projections	74–78	38–47	94–100	217–222
Upper Limb		**Volume 1**		
Anatomy	102–105	60–64	101–111	37–40
Procedural Considerations	106–108	65	112–114	—
Projections (Fingers)	110–119	66–73	115–120	
Projections (Hand)	120–123	74–81	121–124	42–49
Projections (Wrist)	124–131	82–97	125–133	50–54
Projections (Forearm)	132–133	98–100	134–135	55–63
Projections (Elbow)	134–139	101–113	136–142	64–65
Projections (Humerus)	140–145	114–119	143–145	66–75
				76–79
Shoulder Girdle		**Volume 1**		
Anatomy	150–152	122–125	148–152	40–41
Procedural Considerations	153–155	—	153–155	—
Projections (Shoulder)	157–160	126–154	156–164	80–91
Projections (Clavicle)	161–162	157–163	165	94–95
Projections (A–C Joints)	166–167	154–156	166	92–93
Projections (Scapula)	163–165	164–177	168–169	96–98
Lower Limb		**Volume 1**		
Anatomy	170–176	180–185	172–184	99–102
Procedural Considerations	177–181	—	185–188	—
Projections (Toes)	183–187	186–193	189–192	106–109
Projections (Foot)	188–190	194–213	193–196	110–115
Projections (Calcaneus)	191–192	215–227	197–198	116–118
Projections (Ankle)	193–196	228–233	199–203	119–122
Projections (Lower Leg)	197–198	234–239	204–205	123–125
Projections (Knee)	199–203	240–249	206–209	126, 128–131
Projections (Patella)	208–211	256–265	212–216	132–135
Projections (Intercon. fossa)	204–207	250–255	210–211	127
Projections (Femur)	212–215	266–269	217–219	136–139
Pelvic Girdle		**Volume 1**		
Anatomy	220–223	272–275	222–228	103–105
Procedural Considerations	224–227	—	229–232	—
Projections (Pelvis)	229	276–285	234–237	143–154
Projections (Hips)	230–235	286–301	238–241	140–145
Projections (S-I Joints)	236–239	380–383	242–244	201–203

	CORNUELLE & GRONEFELD	BALLINGER	BONTRAGER	EISENBERG
Bony Thorax		**Volume 1**		
Anatomy	248–250	400–403	306–309	155–157
Procedural Considerations	251–253	404–407	310–313	—
Projections (Ribs)	255–259	420–431	318–320	161–167
Projections (Sternum)	260–263	408–413	314–315	158–160
Projections (S-C Joints)	264	414–419	316–317	—
Vertebral Column		**Volume 1**		
Anatomy	268–277	312–323	248–258, 280–284	169–173
Procedural Considerations	278–284	—	260–264, 286–288	—
Projections (Cervical)	286–294	324–355	265–274	175–185
Projections (Thoracic)	296–300	356–363	275–277	186–191
Projections (Lumbar)	301–309	364–379	289–293	192–200
Projections (Sacrum)	310–311	387–389	299, 301	204–206
Projections (Coccyx)	312–313	387–389	300, 302	207–208
Scoliosis/Spinal Fusion	314–315	394–398	294–298	209–211
Skull		**Volume 2**		
Anatomy	320–329	216–227	324–331, 389–393	275–278, 282–283
Procedural Considerations	330–336	233–237	343–348	284–285
Projections (Skull)	338–347	238–269	349–358	286–295, 303–305
Projections (Petrous/Mastoid)	348–353	396–439	402–408	328–336
Facial Bones		**Volume 2**		
Anatomy	358–365	216–232	332–340, 386–387	278–282
Procedural Considerations	365–368	300	360–362	—
Projections (Facial Bones)	376–380, 382–388	301–329	363–365	312–319
Projections (Mandible)	387–391	336–355	373–377	320–325
Projections (TMJs)	392–395	356–367	379–382	326–327
Projections (Sinuses)	370–375	372–393	386–388	297–302
Projections (Orbits)	381	270–285	366	306–311
Urinary System		**Volume 2**		
Anatomy	416–420	152–155	504–510	263
Procedural Considerations	421–427	156–167	511, 514–521	264–265
Projections	429–434	168–192	521–528	266–273
Digestive System		**Volume 2**		
Anatomy	438–449	84–87	412–421, 446–454	213–216
Procedural Considerations	450–458	88–97	422– 431, 455–467	237, 249, 251
Projections	460–481	98–150	435–444, 470–482	232–262
Biliary System		**Volume 2**		
Anatomy	486–489	32–33	484–486	216
Procedural Considerations	490–494	53–57	487–496	—
Projections	496–499	58–80	497–501	223–231
Contrast Media Administration		—		—
	400–412		511–512, 423–424	
Mammography		**Volume 2**		
Anatomy	504–505	460–464	530–533	337–338
Procedural Considerations	506–520	456–459, 465–469	534–537	338–339
Projections	522–525	470–492	537–543	341–346

Continued

► PAGE COMPARISON OF TEXTBOOK BY CORNUELLE & GRONEFELD WITH OTHER COMMONLY USED TEXTS (continued)

	CORNUELLE & GRONEFELD	BALLINGER	BONTRAGER	EISENBERG
Cardiovascular		Volume 2		
Anatomy	528–530	515–521	680–694	366–369
Procedures	531–545	523–587	695–717	370–380
Myelography		Volume 2		
	284	496–505	620–625	360
Arthrography		Volume 1		
	98	488–499	615–619	359

► SAMPLE COURSE OUTLINE: Quarter System

Summer Session

7 weeks, 3 hours per week, 21 hours per quarter (90-minute classes)

WEEK 1

Day 1	Chapter 1	Introduction to Radiography
Day 2	Chapter 1	Introduction to Anatomy & Positioning Terminology

WEEK 2

Day 1	Chapter 2	Anatomy of the Respiratory System
Day 2	Chapter 2	Procedural Considerations & Positioning of the Respiratory System

WEEK 3

Day 1	Chapter 3	Anatomy of the Abdomen
Day 2	Chapter 3	Procedural Considerations & Positioning of the Abdomen

WEEK 4

Day 1	Exam	Chapter 1, 2, 3
	Chapter 4	Musculoskeletal System
Day 2	Chapter 4	Musculoskeletal System/Arthrography

WEEK 5

Day 1	Chapter 5	Anatomy of the Hands & Wrists
Day 2	Chapter 5	Procedural Considerations & Positioning of the Hands & Wrists

WEEK 6

Day 1	Chapter 5	Anatomy of the Forearm, Elbow, & Humerus
Day 2	Chapter 5	Procedural Considerations & Positioning of the Forearm, Elbow, & Humerus

WEEK 7

Day 1	Review	Chapters 1–5
Day 2	Exam	Chapters 1, 2, 3, 4, 5

Fall Quarter

11 weeks, 22 hours per quarter (50-minute classes)

WEEK 1

Day 1	Chapter 6	Anatomy of the Shoulder Girdle
Day 2	Chapter 6	Anatomy of the Shoulder Girdle

WEEK 2

Day 1	Chapter 6	Procedural Considerations & Positioning of the Shoulder Girdle
Day 2	Chapter 6	Procedural Considerations & Positioning of the Shoulder Girdle

WEEK 3

Day 1	Exam	Chapter 6
Day 2	Chapter 7	Anatomy of the Foot & Ankle

WEEK 4

Day 1	Chapter 7	Anatomy of the Foot & Ankle
Day 2	Chapter 7	Procedural Considerations & Positioning of the Foot & Ankle

WEEK 5

Day 1	Chapter 7	Procedural Considerations & Positioning of the Foot & Ankle
Day 2	Chapter 7	Anatomy of the Lower Leg, Knee, & Femur

WEEK 6

Day 1	Chapter 7	Anatomy of the Lower Leg, Knee, & Femur
Day 2	Chapter 7	Procedural Considerations & Positioning of the Lower Leg, Knee, & Femur

WEEK 7

Day 1	Chapter 7	Procedural Considerations & Positioning of the Lower Leg, Knee, & Femur
Day 2	Review	Chapter 7

WEEK 8

Day 1	Exam	Chapter 7
Day 2	Chapter 8	Anatomy of the Pelvic Girdle

WEEK 9

Day 1	Chapter 8	Anatomy of the Pelvic Girdle
Day 2	Chapter 8	Procedural Considerations & Positioning of the Pelvic Girdle

WEEK 10

Day 1	Chapter 8	Procedural Considerations & Positioning of the Pelvic Girdle
Day 2	Exam	Chapter 8

WEEK 11

Day 1	Review	Chapter 6–8
Day 2	Exam	Chapters 6, 7, 8

Winter Quarter

11 weeks, 22 hours per quarter (50-minute classes)

WEEK 1

Day 1	Chapter 9	Anatomy of the Bony Thorax
Day 2	Chapter 9	Procedural Considerations & Positioning of the Bony Thorax

WEEK 2

Day 1	Chapter 9	Procedural Considerations & Positioning of the Bony Thorax
Day 2	Exam	Chapter 9

WEEK 3

Day 1	Chapter 10	Anatomy of the Cervical & Thoracic Spine
Day 2	Chapter 10	Anatomy of the Cervical & Thoracic Spine

WEEK 4

Day 1	Chapter 10	Procedural Considerations & Positioning of the Cervical & Thoracic Spine
Day 2	Chapter 10	Procedural Considerations & Positioning of the Cervical & Thoracic Spine

WEEK 5

Day 1	Chapter 10	Anatomy of the Lumbar Spine, Sacrum, & Coccyx
Day 2	Chapter 10	Anatomy of the Lumbar Spine, Sacrum, & Coccyx

WEEK 6

Day 1	Chapter 10	Procedural Considerations & Positioning of the Lumbar Spine, Sacrum, & Coccyx
Day 2	Chapter 10	Procedural Considerations & Positioning of the Lumbar Spine, Sacrum, & Coccyx

WEEK 7

Day 1	Exam	Chapter 10
Day 2	Chapter 11	Anatomy of the Skull

WEEK 8

Day 1	Chapter 11	Anatomy of the Skull
Day 2	Chapter 11	Procedural Considerations & Positioning of the Skull & Mastoids

WEEK 9

| Day 1 | Chapter 11 | Procedural Considerations & Positioning of the Skull & Mastoids |
| Day 2 | Chapter 12 | Anatomy of the Facial Bones & Paranasal Sinuses |

WEEK 10

| Day 1 | Chapter 12 | Anatomy of the Facial Bones & Paranasal Sinuses |
| Day 2 | Chapter 12 | Procedural Considerations & Positioning of the Facial Bones & Paranasal Sinuses |

WEEK 11

| Day 1 | Chapter 12 | Procedural Considerations & Positioning of the Facial Bones & Paranasal Sinuses |
| Day 2 | Exam | Chapters 9, 10, 11, 12 |

Spring Quarter

11 weeks, 22 hours per quarter (50-minute classes)

WEEK 1

| Day 1 | Chapter 13 | Introduction to Contrast Studies |
| Day 2 | Chapter 13 | Contrast Media & Reactions |

WEEK 2

| Day 1 | Chapter 14 | Anatomy of the Urinary System |
| Day 2 | Chapter 14 | Procedural Considerations of the Urinary System |

WEEK 3

| Day 1 | Chapter 14 | Positioning of the Urinary System |
| Day 2 | Exam | Chapters 13, 14 |

WEEK 4

| Day 1 | Chapter 15 | Anatomy of the Gastrointestinal System |
| Day 2 | Chapter 15 | Anatomy of the Gastrointestinal System |

WEEK 5

| Day 1 | Chapter 15 | Procedural Considerations for Radiography of the Upper & Lower Gastrointestinal Tract |
| Day 2 | Chapter 15 | Positioning of the Upper Gastrointestinal Tract |

WEEK 6

| Day 1 | Chapter 15 | Positioning of the Lower Gastrointestinal Tract |
| Day 2 | Exam | Chapter 15 |

WEEK 7

| Day 1 | Chapter 16 | Anatomy of the Biliary System |
| Day 2 | Chapter 16 | Procedural Considerations & Positioning of the Biliary System |

WEEK 8

| Day 1 | Chapter 17 | Anatomy of the Breast |
| Day 2 | Chapter 17 | Procedural Considerations for Mammography |

WEEK 9

| Day 1 | Chapter 17 | Mammography |
| Day 2 | Exam | Chapters 16, 17 |

WEEK 10

| Day 1 | Chapter 18 | Cardiovascular System |
| Day 2 | Chapter 18 | Cardiovascular System |

WEEK 11

| Day 1 | Chapter 18 | Cardiovascular System/Lymphangiography |
| Day 2 | Exam | Chapters 13, 14, 15, 16, 17, 18 |

► SAMPLE COURSE OUTLINE: Semester System

Summer Session

5 weeks, 3 hours per week, 15 hours (90-minute classes)

WEEK 1

| Day 1 | Chapter 1 | Professional Ethics |
| Day 2 | Chapter 1 | Communication |

WEEK 2

| Day 1 | Chapter 1 | Infection Control |
| Day 2 | Chapter 1 | Introduction to Anatomy & Procedural Considerations |

WEEK 3

| Day 1 | Chapter 1 | Technical Considerations & Radiation Protection |
| Day 2 | Chapter 1 | Image Evaluation & Film Critique |

WEEK 4

| Day 1 | Chapter 2 | Anatomy of the Respiratory System |
| Day 2 | Chapter 2 | Procedural Considerations of the Respiratory System |

WEEK 5

| Day 1 | Chapter 2 | Positioning of the Respiratory System |
| Day 2 | Exam | Chapters 1, 2 |

Fall Semester

16 weeks, 3 hours per week (50-minute classes)

WEEK 1

Day 1	Course Overview	
Day 2	Chapter 3	Anatomy of the Abdomen
Day 3	Chapter 3	Procedural Considerations for the Abdomen

WEEK 2

Day 1	Chapter 3	Positioning of the Abdomen
Day 2	Chapter 4	Musculoskeletal System
Day 3	Chapter 4	Musculoskeletal System

WEEK 3

Day 1	Labor Day Holiday	
Day 2	Chapter 5	Anatomy of the Hands & Wrists
Day 3	Chapter 5	Anatomy of the Hands & Wrists

WEEK 4

Day 1	Chapter 5	Procedural Considerations & Positioning of the Hands & Wrists
Day 2	Chapter 5	Procedural Considerations & Positioning of the Hands & Wrists
Day 3	Exam	Chapters 3, 4, 5

WEEK 5

Day 1	Chapter 5	Anatomy of the Forearm, Elbow, & Humerus
Day 2	Chapter 5	Anatomy of the Forearm, Elbow, & Humerus
Day 3	Chapter 5	Procedural Considerations & Positioning of the Forearm, Elbow, & Humerus

WEEK 6

Day 1	Chapter 5	Procedural Considerations & Positioning of the Forearm, Elbow, & Humerus
Day 2	Chapter 6	Anatomy of the Shoulder Girdle
Day 3	Chapter 6	Procedural Considerations of the Shoulder Girdle

WEEK 7

Day 1	Chapter 6	Positioning of the Shoulder Girdle
Day 2	Exam	Chapters 5, 6
Day 3	Chapter 7	Anatomy of the Foot & Ankle

WEEK 8

Day 1	Chapter 7	Anatomy of the Foot & Ankle
Day 2	Chapter 7	Procedural Considerations of the Foot & Ankle
Day 3	Chapter 7	Positioning of the Foot & Ankle

WEEK 9

Day 1	Chapter 7	Positioning of the Foot & Ankle
Day 2	Chapter 7	Anatomy of the Lower Leg, Knee, & Femur
Day 3	Chapter 7	Anatomy of the Lower Leg, Knee, & Femur

WEEK 10

Day 1	Chapter 7	Procedural Considerations of the Lower Leg, Knee, & Femur
Day 2	Chapter 7	Positioning of the Lower Leg, Knee, & Femur
Day 3	Chapter 7	Positioning of the Lower Leg, Knee, & Femur

WEEK 11

Day 1	Exam	Chapter 7
Day 2	Chapter 8	Anatomy of the Pelvic Girdle
Day 3	Chapter 8	Anatomy of the Pelvic Girdle

WEEK 12

Day 1	Chapter 8	Procedural Considerations of the Pelvic Girdle
Day 2	Chapter 8	Positioning of the Pelvic Girdle
Day 3	Chapter 9	Anatomy of the Bony Thorax

WEEK 13

Day 1	Chapter 9	Procedural Considerations of the Bony Thorax
Day 2	Chapter 9	Positioning of the Bony Thorax
Day 3	Chapter 10	Anatomy of the Cervical & Thoracic Spine

WEEK 14

Day 1	Chapter 10	Anatomy of the Cervical & Thoracic Spine
Day 2	Thanksgiving Holiday	
Day 3	Thanksgiving Holiday	

WEEK 15

Day 1	Chapter 10	Procedural Considerations of the Cervical & Thoracic Spine
Day 2	Chapter 10	Procedural Considerations of the Cervical & Thoracic Spine
Day 3	Chapter 10	Positioning of the Cervical & Thoracic Spine

WEEK 16

Day 1	Chapter 10	Positioning of the Cervical & Thoracic Spine
Day 2	Exam	Chapters 8, 9, 10
Day 3	Review for Final Exam	

SCHEDULED FINAL EXAM

Comprehensive Final

Spring Semester

16 weeks, 3 hours per week (50-minute classes)

WEEK 1

Day 1	Course Overview	
Day 2	Chapter 10	Anatomy of the Lumbar Spine, Sacrum, & Coccyx
Day 3	Chapter 10	Procedural Considerations & Positioning of the Lumbar Spine, Sacrum, & Coccyx

WEEK 2

Day 1	Martin Luther King Holiday	
Day 2	Chapter 10	Procedural Considerations & Positioning of the Lumbar Spine, Sacrum, & Coccyx
Day 3	Chapter 11	Introduction to Anatomy of the Skull

WEEK 3

Day 1	Chapter 11	Anatomy of the Skull
Day 2	Chapter 11	Anatomy of the Petrous Portions
Day 3	Chapter 11	Anatomy of the Petrous Portions

WEEK 4

Day 1	Chapter 11	Positioning Considerations of the Skull
Day 2	Chapter 11	Positioning Considerations of the Petrous Portions
Day 3	Chapter 11	Positioning of the Skull

WEEK 5

Day 1	Chapter 11	Positioning of the Petrous Portions
Day 2	Exam	Chapters 10, 11
Day 3	Chapter 12	Anatomy of the Facial Bones

WEEK 6

Day 1	Chapter 12	Anatomy of the Facial Bones
Day 2	Chapter 12	Anatomy of the Facial Bones
Day 3	Chapter 12	Anatomy of the Facial Bones

WEEK 7

Day 1	Presidents Day	
Day 2	Chapter 12	Anatomy of the Paranasal Sinuses
Day 3	Chapter 12	Procedural Considerations & Positioning of the Sinuses

WEEK 8

Day 1	Chapter 12	Positioning of the Paranasal Sinuses
Day 2	Chapter 12	Procedural Considerations & Positioning of the Facial Bones
Day 3	Chapter 12	Procedural Considerations & Positioning of the Facial Bones

WEEK 9

Day 1	Chapter 12	Procedural Considerations & Positioning of the Facial Bones
Day 2	Chapter 12	Procedural Considerations & Positioning of the Facial Bones
Day 3	Exam	Chapter 12

WEEK 10

Spring Break

WEEK 11

Day 1	Chapter 13	Introduction to Contrast Studies
Day 2	Chapter 13	Contrast Media Reactions
Day 3	Chapter 14	Anatomy of the Urinary System

WEEK 12

Day 1	Chapter 14	Anatomy of the Urinary System
Day 2	Chapter 14	Anatomy of the Urinary System
Day 3	Chapter 14	Procedural Considerations of the Urinary System

WEEK 13

Day 1	Chapter 14	Positioning of the Urinary System
Day 2	Exam	Chapters 13, 14
Day 3	Chapter 15	Anatomy of the Gastrointestinal System

WEEK 14

Day 1	Chapter 15	Anatomy of the Gastrointestinal System
Day 2	Chapter 15	Procedural Considerations for Radiography of the Upper Gastrointestinal Tract
Day 3	Chapter 15	Procedural Considerations for Radiography of the Lower Gastrointestinal Tract

WEEK 15

Day 1	Chapter 15	Positioning of the Upper Gastrointestinal Tract
Day 2	Chapter 15	Positioning of the Lower Gastrointestinal Tract
Day 3	Chapter 16	Anatomy of the Biliary System

WEEK 16

Day 1	Chapter 16	Procedural Considerations & Positioning of the Biliary System
Day 2	Exam	Chapters 15, 16
Day 3	Review	

SCHEDULED FINAL EXAM

Comprehensive Final

Fall Semester of Second Year

Special Radiographic Equipment and Procedures Class
Chapter 17   Mammography 3–4 hours
Chapter 18   Cardiovascular Studies   6–7 hours

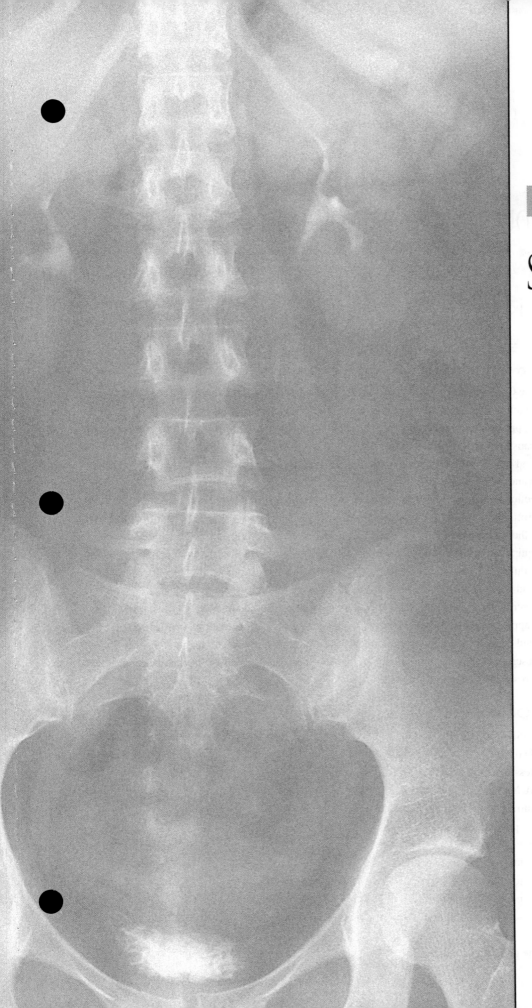

2

SECTION

1 INTRODUCTION TO RADIOGRAPHY

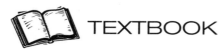 TEXTBOOK

Objectives

Following the completion of this chapter, the student will be able to:

1. Discuss the Code of Ethics and professionalism as they relate to the radiologic technologist.
2. Describe factors relative to effective communication with patients of all ages.
3. Describe appropriate infection-control procedures and the radiographer's role in prevention of disease transmission.
4. Identify and describe the four basic types of body habitus and explain how they may affect patient centering and positioning.
5. Define sectional anatomy and differentiate between sagittal, coronal, and transverse/axial images.
6. Define terminology related to patient/part positioning.
7. Describe the appropriate steps for completion of a radiographic examination to include room/patient/equipment preparation, appropriate use of lead identification markers, and post-examination procedure.
8. Identify and describe the factors that contribute to image quality.
9. Briefly describe the radiographic and accessory equipment used in the radiology department.
10. Describe appropriate methods of radiation protection for the radiographer and patient.
11. Identify and describe five general components of a systemic film evaluation.
12. Briefly describe computed tomography, diagnostic medical sonography, nuclear medicine, and magnetic resonance imaging.

Chapter Outline

I. PROFESSIONAL ETHICS
   A. Code of Ethics
   B. Professionalism
II. COMMUNICATION & PATIENT CARE
   A. Communicating with the Patient
      1. the pediatric patient
         a. neonates
         b. infants
         c. toddlers
         d. preschool children
         e. school-age children
         f. adolescents
      2. the geriatric patient

III. INFECTION CONTROL
    A. Universal Precautions
    B. Isolation Procedures
IV. INTRODUCTION TO ANATOMY
    A. Body Habitus
    B. Sectional Anatomy
V. PROCEDURAL CONSIDERATIONS
    A. General Positioning Terminology
    B. Guidelines for Use of Lead Markers
    C. Procedural Protocol
VI. TECHNICAL CONSIDERATIONS
    A. Image Characteristics
        1. visibility qualities
            a. radiographic density
            b. radiographic contrast
                (1) subject contrast
                (2) film contrast
        2. geometric qualities
            a. recorded detail (sharpness)
            b. magnification
            c. shape distortion
    B. Equipment Considerations
        1. film screen combinations
        2. radiographic grids
        3. automatic exposure control
    C. Radiographic Equipment
        1. radiographic tables
        2. upright wall units
        3. fluoroscopic equipment
        4. tomographic equipment
        5. mobile equipment
        6. ancillary equipment
VII. RADIATION PROTECTION
    A. Patient Protection
        1. eliminate the need for repeat radiographs
        2. optimum selection of exposure factors
        3. filtration
        4. appropriate selection of image receptors
        5. collimation
        6. protective shielding
        7. managing the potentially pregnant patient
    B. Personnel Protection
        1. the pregnant radiographer
VIII. IMAGE EVALUATION & FILM CRITIQUE
    A. Film Display
    B. Systemic Evaluation
        1. film identification

2. radiation protection
3. patient positioning
4. radiographic quality
5. anatomy

IX. RELATED IMAGING MODALITIES
   A. Computed Tomography
   B. Diagnostic Medical Sonography (Ultrasound)
   C. Nuclear Medicine
   D. Magnetic Resonance Imaging
X. SUMMARY
XI. CRITICAL THINKING & APPLICATION QUESTIONS
XII. FILM CRITIQUE

► SAMPLE 50-MINUTE LESSON

PREPARATION STEP   ESTIMATED TIME—10 MINUTES

A. Assemble teaching aids
   1. Overhead projector
   2. Overhead transparencies
      a. included in *Instructor's Resource Manual*
   3. Skeleton
   4. Anatomy model
   5. Radiographs
B. Introduce topics of the language of radiography. Lecture will include Chapter Objectives 4, 5, & 6.
C. Opening discussion
   1. It is imperative that you learn the material in this chapter very well. The terms presented in this Introduction to Anatomy lesson are very basic and many other terms and concepts will be based on them.
   2. Practice the basic positions until you can do them correctly in a timely manner.

PRESENTATION STEP   ESTIMATED TIME—40 MINUTES

TEACHING OUTLINE	TEACHING AIDS & METHODS
I. Introduction to Anatomy	
A. Body Habitus	*Transparency of body habitus*
1. hypersthenic	*characteristics*
a. 5% of population	
b. broad massive	
c. short thoracic cavity	
d. stomach high and horizontal	*Explain etiology of habitus terms*
2. sthenic	*sthenic = active, strong*
a. 50% of population	
b. modification of hypersthenic	
3. hyposthenic	
a. 35% of population	*Chest radiographs & UGIs that*
b. thorax is longer	*demonstrate body habitus*
c. stomach lower and closer to midline	

        4. asthenic
          a. 10% of population
          b. thorax is narrow & shallow
          c. stomach low, vertical, near midline

Point out various body habitus
among students

B. Sectional Anatomy
    1. must be able to visualize anatomy in
       various different planes
    2. must know anatomy extremely well to be
       able to do this
    3. must know the relationship of all structures
       in the body (ie, anterior/posterior, medial/lateral
       and superior/inferior)

C. Procedural Considerations
    1. in most cases must obtain two
       projections/positions 90° apart
       a. foreign body
       b. alignment of fracture

Two radiographs 90° apart showing
foreign body or alignment

    2. to demonstrate joints obtain three
       projections/positions

D. General Positioning Terminology
    1. anatomic position and planes

Transparencies of planes
& positions

       a. anatomic position
       b. coronal
         (1) midcoronal/midaxillary
       c. sagittal
         (1) midsagittal/medial
       d. transverse/horizontal
       e. oblique
    2. positions

Demonstrate positions using
anatomy model & skeleton

       a. supine (dorsal recumbent)
       b. prone (ventral recumbent)
       c. right & left lateral recumbent
       d. oblique
         (1) LPO
         (2) RPO
         (3) LAO
         (4) RAO
       e. decubitus
         (1) right & left lateral decubitus
         (2) dorsal decubitus
         (3) ventral decubitus
       f. Trendelenburg
       g. Fowler's
       h. Sim's
    3. projection terminology
       a. projection
         (1) AP
         (2) PA
         (3) lateral
         (4) tangential
         (5) axial
       b. view
    4. directional/relationship terminology
       a. anterior/ventral
       b. posterior/dorsal

        c. medial/mesial

        d. lateral

        e. proximal

        f. distal

        g. cephalad/cephalic/cranial/superior

        h. caudad/caudal/inferior

    5. part/body movement

        a. flexion

           (1) hyperflexion

        b. extension

           (1) hyperextension

        c. dorsiflexion

        d. inversion

        e. eversion

        f. abduction

        g. adduction

        h. pronation

        i. supination

        j. rotation

        k. tilt

APPLICATION STEP   ESTIMATED TIME—2 HOURS

Study Assignment

A. Continue reading Chapter 1 in the text.

B. Continue Chapter 1 in the *Applications Manual.*

C. Study the radiographs for this chapter. Be sure you can differentiate body habitus, body planes, body positions, and projections.

D. Observe the different body types of the people you come in contact with, and ascertain which type habitus they exhibit.

TESTING STEP

Questions on this material will be included in exam given at end of this chapter.

► EXAM QUESTIONS

Multiple Choice

1. The lungs on the radiograph you are critiquing are broader superiorly and narrower at the bases. They are long and narrow. Which body type is the patient?

    A. hypersthenic

    B. sthenic

    C. hyposthenic

    D. asthenic

2. What is/are the reason(s) two projections/positions 90° apart are obtained for most radiographic exams?

    1. for localization of foreign objects

    2. to assess fracture alignment

3. many body parts are superimposed on a two-dimensional radiograph
   A. 1 only
   B. 2 only
   C. 2 and 3 only
   D. 1, 2, and 3

3. What information must be included in the patient identification area of the radiograph?
   1. name of exam performed
   2. patient name or x-ray number
   3. facility name
   A. 1 only
   B. 2 only
   C. 2 and 3 only
   D. 1, 2, and 3

4. What is the purpose of increasing the SID when there is a large OID?
   A. an increase in SID compensates for a large OID and reduces magnification
   B. an increase in SID compensates for the decreased technique necessary when there is a large OID
   C. the SID is increased to increase the size of the structure on the radiograph
   D. the SID is increased to eliminate the shape distortion caused by the OID

5. Why is a radiographic grid necessary when obtaining a radiograph of a body part measuring 10 cm or more?
   A. it decreases the amount of radiation to the patient
   B. is absorbs scatter radiation exiting the patient
   C. it decreases contrast on the resulting radiograph
   D. it increases the density on the resulting radiograph

6. What is the name of the device that measures the amount of radiation that reaches the film and automatically ends the exposure when the correct amount is measured?
   A. radiographic grid
   B. focal spot
   C. AEC
   D. Bucky mechanism

7. How should a chest radiograph be displayed on the viewbox?
   A. the patient's right side should be on your right side whether the projection was an AP or PA
   B. the patient's right side should be on your left side whether the projection was an AP or PA
   C. if it is a PA chest the patient's right side should be on your right side
   D. if it is an AP chest the patient's left side should be on your left side

8. As you are giving patient preparation instructions to your next patient you notice that his chest is very broad and massive. What body habitus is this individual?
   A. hypersthenic
   B. sthenic
   C. hyposthenic
   D. asthenic

9. How would you describe a patient who is in the LPO position?
   A. the patient's left posterior side is closest to the table or upright Bucky
   B. the patient's left anterior side is closest to the table or upright Bucky

C. the patient's left posterior side is farthest away from the table or upright Bucky

D. the patient is lying on the left side in a lateral position

10. How would you describe a patient who is in the right lateral recumbent position?

A. standing at the upright Bucky with the right side closest to the board

B. standing at the upright Bucky with the left side closest to the board

C. lying down on the table with the right side closest to the cassette which is in the Bucky

D. lying down on the table with the left side closest to the cassette which is in the Bucky

11. In radiographic terminology what does the positioning term *decubitus* signify?

A. the patient is standing up at the upright Bucky and the central ray is horizontal and parallel to the floor

B. the patient is standing up at the upright Bucky and the central ray is vertical and parallel to the Bucky

C. the patient is lying on the table and the central ray is perpendicular to the table

D. the patient is lying on the table and the central ray is horizontal and parallel to the floor

12. In radiographic terminology what does the positioning term *ventral decubitus* signify?

A. the patient is lying on the table in a supine position and the central ray is horizontal and parallel to the floor

B. the patient is lying on the table in a prone position and the central ray is horizontal and parallel to the floor

C. the patient is lying on his/her left side and the central ray enters the patient's ventral side first

D. the patient is lying on his/her right side and the central ray enters the patient's ventral side first

13. The patient is standing at the upright Bucky with his/her ventral side closest to the film. Describe the projection of the central ray.

A. anteroposterior

B. posteroanterior

C. tangential

D. axial

14. The hand is _____ to the shoulder.

A. lateral

B. medial

C. proximal

D. distal

15. An axial central ray projecting toward the head of the patient is termed a _____ angle.

A. lateral

B. medial

C. cephalic

D. caudal

Answer Key

1. D	4. A	7. B	10. C	13. B
2. D	5. B	8. A	11. D	14. D
3. C	6. C	9. A	12. B	15. C

APPLICATIONS MANUAL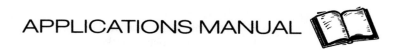

ANSWER KEY FOR STUDY QUESTIONS ◄

1. Code of Ethics
2. Attitudes are a set of beliefs that an individual holds. They can lead to biases and/or discrimination, which can affect one's behavior, thus impacting patient care. A radiographer's values and attitudes can conflict with those of a patient.
3. A 4-year-old child is considered to be preschool age. Because he or she is able to communicate verbally and has a basic understanding, he or she should be given an explanation of the examination. The radiographer can show him/her the equipment to help alleviate any fears. The radiographer should praise the child's performance during the examination.
4. Nosocomial refers to a hospital-acquired infection. The patient was exposed to the sick radiographer and contracted the illness while in the hospital.
5. Whenever there is a possibility of splashes or droplets of blood or body fluid touching the face or eyes.
6. You are responsible for positioning the patient. You will handle the cassette only after it has been placed in a protective plastic cover. You will not manipulate the radiographic equipment.
7. Body habitus
8. Two projections 90° apart from each other are required for localization of foreign objects.
9. Sthenic
10. Midcoronal or midaxillary
11. Sagittal
12. Ventral
13. Toward
14. Distal
15. Proximal
16. Medial
17. Distal
18. Distal
19. Lateral
20. Lateral
21. Eversion
22. Adduction
23. Flexion
24. Extension
25. Pronation
26. Rotation
27. Tilt
28. Supination
29. Away from
30. Inversion
31. Left lateral
32. Oblique
33. The anterior or palmar surface
34. Projection
35. Supine
36. Trendelenburg
37. Tangential
38. A projection in which the CR passes from the posterior to the anterior aspect of the body
39. Dorsal decubitus

40. Sim's position
41. Right anterior oblique (RAO)
42. Left posterior oblique (RPO)
43. Fowler's
44. Patient name and/or x-ray number, patient age or date of birth, date and time of the examination, name of patient's physician, and the name of the facility
45. Left marker on the cassette because you are doing a left lateral projection. The side closest to the film should always be marked on a lateral projection.
46. Radiographic density
47. SID is the source-image distance, which is the distance between the x-ray tube and the image receptor (film).
48. kVp; mAs
49. Radiographic contrast
50. High
51. High
52. There is a direct relationship between magnification and OID. Magnification is increased since OID is increased.
53. Cassette
54. Inside the cassette (may be only on one or on both sides)
55. Slow; fast
56. Grid
57. The photocells are selected to correspond to the centering of the anatomy of interest
58. Keep radiation exposures *as low as reasonably achievable*
59. Floating
60. Fluoroscopic
61. C-arm
62. Tomography
63. Calipers
64. Positioning sponges
65. Lead
66. Genetic
67. Collimation
68. Time, distance, and shielding
69. Radiographic images should be displayed as if looking at the front of the patient. On the PA projection, the patient's right side should be on the radiographer's left side.
70. CT: computed tomography; MRI: magnetic resonance imaging
71. Computed tomography (CT)
72. Diagnostic medical sonography (ultrasound)
73. Radio
74. Radionuclide
75. Film badge, thermoluminescent dosimeter (TLD), or pocket ionization chamber

ANSWER KEY FOR CROSSWORD PUZZLE ◄

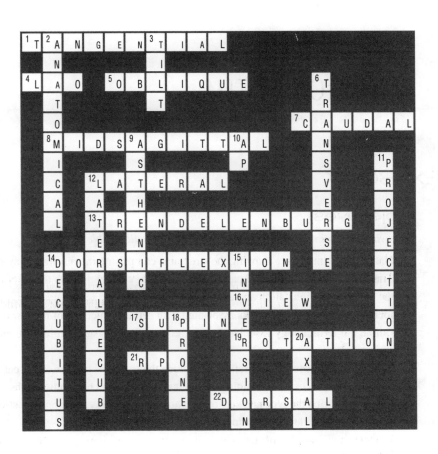

ACROSS

1. tangential
4. LAO
5. oblique
7. caudal
8. midsagittal
12. lateral
13. Trendelenburg
14. dorsiflexion
16. view
17. supine
19. rotation
21. RPO
22. dorsal

DOWN

2. anatomical
3. tilt
6. transverse
9. asthenic
10. AP
11. projection
12. lateral decub
14. decubitus
15. inversion
18. prone
20. axial

2 RESPIRATORY SYSTEM

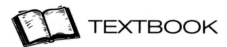 TEXTBOOK

Objectives

Following the completion of this chapter, the student will be able to:

1. Name and identify on a drawing the structures comprising the respiratory system.
2. Trace the path of oxygen and carbon dioxide as they travel through the respiratory system during the processes of inhalation and exhalation.
3. Identify the skeletal landmarks associated with certain structures of the respiratory system.
4. Define the terminology associated with the respiratory system, to include anatomy, procedures, and pathology.
5. Describe the process of respiration, to include the transit of oxygen to the cells of the body.
6. Describe the process for obtaining routine and nonroutine chest radiographs.
7. List and describe the type and size of film holder, central ray location, and structures best demonstrated on routine and nonroutine projections of the chest.
8. Evaluate radiographs of the chest in terms of positioning, centering, image quality, and radiographic anatomy.
9. Simulate the positioning for routine and nonroutine projections of the chest on another student or phantom.
10. Discuss the technical and equipment considerations involved in producing optimum radiographs of the chest.
11. Discuss the positioning and technique modifications necessary when performing chest radiography on children and using a mobile unit at the patient's bedside.
12. Identify technical changes necessary to compensate for various pathologic conditions.
13. Identify alternative methods of imaging the chest.

Chapter Outline

    I. ANATOMY OF THE RESPIRATORY SYSTEM
        A. Pharynx
            1. nasopharynx
            2. oropharynx
            3. laryngopharynx
        B. Larynx
        C. Trachea
        D. Bronchi
        E. Alveoli

► SAMPLE 50-MINUTE LESSON

PREPARATION STEP   ESTIMATED TIME—10 MINUTES

A. Assemble teaching aids
1. Overhead projector
2. Overhead transparencies
   a. included in Instructor's Resource Manual
   b. trace drawings from Applications Manual on clear radiographic film
3. Anatomy model
4. Radiographs
B. Introduce topic of anatomy and positioning of the respiratory system
C. Opening discussion
1. You will most likely perform hundreds of chest x-rays in your career as a Radiologic Technologist. It is important to remember that each CXR is performed on an unique person. Even though you will become very familiar with this procedure, remember that it may be the first x-ray the patient has ever had. Be sure your directions to the patient are clear and concise.
2. The CXR can be a valuable diagnostic tool if it is performed correctly. Strive to always produce excellent radiographs as this will ultimately benefit the patient.

PRESENTATION STEP   ESTIMATED TIME—40 MINUTES

TEACHING OUTLINE	TEACHING AIDS & METHODS
I. Respiratory system	
A. Pharynx	
B. Trachea	
C. Bronchi	*Point out parts on anatomic model*
D. Lungs	
II. Pharynx	
A. Functions in Both the Respiratory and Digestive Systems	
1. nasopharynx	*Point out parts on radiograph*
a. posterior to two nasal cavities	
b. superior and posterior to soft palate	
2. oropharynx	
a. posterior to mouth	*Use overhead transparencies when*
3. laryngopharynx	*appropriate*
a. inferior to epiglottis	
III. Larynx	
A. Anterior Portion of Neck Between C-3 and C-6	
B. 5 cm Long	
C. Composed of Nine Cartilages	
1. thyroid cartilage—Adam's Apple	
a. largest	
b. located at C-5	
2. cricoid cartilage	
a. tracheostomies performed just below this point	
D. Epiglottis	
1. top of larynx	
2. leaf-shaped flap forms lid over glottis	

E. Glottis
   1. slit-like opening between horizontal folds
   2. false vocal cords—upper folds
   3. true vocal cords—lower folds

IV. Trachea
   A. 2–2.5 cm in Diameter
   B. 10–11 cm Long
   C. Anterior to Esophagus
   D. Located in Mediastinum
   E. Extends from C-6 to T4–5
   F. 16–20 C-Shaped Rings
      1. open portion of ring is posterior

V. Bronchi
   A. Trachea Bifurcates at T-4 or T-5 into Right and Left
   B. Primary Bronchi
      1. carina
         a. ridge of cartilage found at lower end of trachea
            where it branches
   C. Right Primary Bronchus
      1. conveys air into and out of right lung
      2. wider, shorter, more vertical
      3. foreign body aspiration most likely
      4. branches into three secondary bronchi
         a. secondary bronchi branch into bronchioles
   D. Left Primary Bronchus
      1. conveys air into and out of left lung
      2. narrower, longer, less vertical
      3. branches into two secondary bronchi
         a. secondary bronchi branch into bronchioles

VI. Alveoli
   A. Clusters of Small Air Sacs
   B. Thin Walls in Close Contact With Capillaries
   C. Functional Units Within Lungs Where Exchange of O_2 and
      CO_2 Between Alveoli and Surrounding Capillaries Occurs

VII. Lungs
   A. Apex
   B. Base
   C. Costal Surface
      1. lies against ribs
   D. Hilum
   E. Costophrenic Angles
   F. Cardiac Notch/Angle
      1. inferior, medial aspect of left lung
      2. concavity caused by border of heart resting against lung
   G. Right Lung
      1. shorter and broader due to liver
      2. divided into three lobes
   H. Left Lung
      1. longer and narrower
      2. divided into two lobes
   I. Pleura
      1. membranous covering of lungs and thoracic cavity
      2. double fold of serous membrane
         a. visceral pleura covers lungs
         b. parietal pleura lines thoracic cavity

(1) small space between contains
    lubricating fluid
    (a) location of pneumothorax or
        pleural effusion
J. Parenchyma
    1. spongy, elastic material that makes up
       composition of lungs
VIII. Mediastinum
    A. Area Between Lungs
    B. Heart
    C. Great Vessels
        1. aorta, superior & inferior vena cava, pul-
           monary arteries, pulmonary veins
    D. Thymus Gland
    E. Trachea
    F. Esophagus
IX. Diaphragm
    A. Separates Thoracic and Abdominal Cavities
    B. Hemidiaphragm
        1. one under each lung

APPLICATION STEP   ESTIMATED TIME—2 HOURS

Study Assignment

A. Read Chapter 2 in the text.
B. Find all the anatomy discussed on the anatomic model.
C. Find all the anatomy discussed on the chest radiographs.
D. Begin Chapter 2 in the *Applications Manual*.

TESTING STEP

Questions on this material will be included in exam given at end of Chapter 2.

► EXAM QUESTIONS

Matching

1. _____ Hilus   A. broad lower portion of the lung

2. _____ Apex   B. double-walled membranous sac enclosing the heart

3. _____ Base of the lungs   C. muscular structure separating thoracic and abdominal
                                        cavities

4. _____ Diaphragm   D. central area of lungs where bronchi enter

5. _____ Costophrenic angles   E. lateral portion of lungs

6. _____ Pleura   F. outermost corners of base of lung

                                    G. part of lung around the heart

                                    H. upper area of lung above clavicles

Multiple Choice

7. What is the purpose of rolling the shoulders forward when performing a PA upright chest radiograph?
    A. to ensure that there is no rotation
    B. to remove the scapulae from the lung field
    C. to allow the patient to be in a comfortable position
    D. to project the clavicles above the lung field

8. Why is it important to perform chest x-rays with the patient in an upright position whenever possible?
    1. to assist the diaphragm in its downward movement
    2. to allow for visualization of fluid levels
    3. to allow for better expansion of the lungs
        A. 1 only
        B. 1 and 2 only
        C. 2 and 3 only
        D. 1, 2, and 3

9. What is the best criterion for determining on a PA chest radiograph whether or not the patient took in a deep inspiration?
    A. the diaphragm will be outlined under the lungs
    B. ten posterior ribs will be seen within the lung field
    C. the heart will appear very enlarged
    D. the trachea will be filled with air

10. When a person aspirates a foreign body where is it most likely to go?
    A. down the right primary bronchus
    B. down the left primary bronchus
    C. it will be lodged at the carina
    D. the direction is impossible to predict

11. What are the correct breathing instructions for a PA and lateral chest radiograph?
    A. "take in a deep breath and hold it"
    B. "take in a breath, blow it all the way out and hold it"
    C. "take in a deep breath, blow it out, take in another deep breath and hold it"
    D. "slowly take in a deep breath"

12. Which radiographic projection of the chest may be requested to better demonstrate the apices of the lungs?
    A. PA
    B. AP
    C. lordotic
    D. oblique

13. Which radiographic projection of the chest may be requested to evaluate suspicious areas seen on previous chest radiographs or to evaluate the heart?
    A. PA
    B. AP
    C. lordotic
    D. oblique

14. Expiration PA chest radiographs are sometimes requested to rule out
   A. pneumonia
   B. pneumothorax
   C. emphysema
   D. cardiomegaly

Answer Key

1. D	4. C	7. B	10. A	13. D
2. H	5. F	8. D	11. C	14. B
3. A	6. B	9. B	12. C	

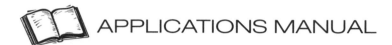

APPLICATIONS MANUAL

▶ DRAWINGS

The students should color each anatomic part a different color (ie. heart one color, lungs another color). The act of coloring causes them to pay very close attention to all the parts of the drawing. The drawings were done by a Radiologic Technologist and are quite accurate. Labeling the parts is also very important for the student to become proficient in this most basic part of anatomy and positioning. Many students who were doubtful about the benefits of "coloring pictures" felt that they could visualize the anatomy much better after they were finished.

▶ ANSWER KEY FOR STUDY QUESTIONS

1. A. pharynx   C. bronchi
   B. trachea   D. right & left lungs
2. Warm and moisten
3. Pharynx
4. Epiglottis
5. Hyoid
6. Larynx
7. Oropharynx
8. Cricoid
9. Thyroid cartilage or Adam's apple
10. 4 in. (10–11 cm); anterior
11. 16–20 C-shaped rings of cartilage
12. T-5; primary bronchi
13. Carina
14. The right primary bronchus is wider, shorter, and more vertical than the left primary bronchus.
15. 3; 2 (to correspond respectively with the number of lobes in each lung)
16. Bronchioles are very small branches of the bronchi
17. Alveoli
18. Apex
19. Alveoli
20. Base
21. Hila (or hili)
22. Costophrenic angles

23. Fissures
24. Pleura; visceral pleura; parietal pleura
25. Pulmonary veins
26. Diaphragm
27. Parenchyma
28. Mediastinum
29. Capillaries
30. 10–20
31. Breathing; difficult or painful breathing
32. This information can assist the radiologist in making an accurate diagnosis. It can also aid the radiographer in positioning and setting technical factors. For example, if the patient had his left lung removed, the radiographer would want to take a right lateral projection and would also need to decrease density if setting the technique manually.
33. Inferiorly
34. The scapulae are in the lung fields
35. 10
36. If the chin is not elevated, it will create an artifact in the apices of the lungs
37. Sternoclavicular joints
38. High
39. High
40. 100–150 kVp
41. A short time will minimize breathing and heart motion.
42. 72 in.
43. The center cell
44. Deep inspiration—take in a deep breath, exhale, take in another deep breath and hold it
45. Lateral upper airway (soft tissue neck)
46. Left lateral decubitus
47. Left lateral decubitus
48. Apices of the lungs
49. AP upper airway
50. Place the cassette under the patient's chest. Angle the central ray 20° and direct it to a point 2 in. below mid-sternum.
51. AP
52. Use the following conversion factor: 0.25 × adult mAs
53. You must have a caudal angle since the patient is learning back in a semi-erect position. Adjust the degree of the central ray until it is directed perpendicular to the patient's coronal plane.
54. The central ray was not perpendicular to the patient's coronal plane. The degree of the caudal angle must be increased.
55. Destructive
56. A
57. A
58. D
59. A
60. D
61. A
62. D
63. T6–7 (inferior angle of the scapula)
64. The posterior ribs are superimposed; the lung fields are superimposed; the sternum and thoracic spine are demonstrated in a lateral position.
65. RAO (right anterior oblique)
66. Left
67. The level of the thyroid cartilage
68. Left
69. C-3 through T-5

70. False; although chest radiography may be done without a grid, a grid is usually used to cut down on scatter and because the chest measures greater than 10 cm.
71. True
72. False; the esophagus is present in the mediastinum but is not visible without the aid of contrast media.
73. True
74. True
75.

Projection	CR Angle/ Angle of Part	Centering Point	Film Size	Structures Seen
Lateral upper airway	Horizontal beam	1 in. superior to level of suprasternal notch	10 × 12 in. lw	Air-filled larynx and trachea anterior to the spine; epiglottis
Left anterior oblique	Horizontal beam Mid-sagittal plane rotated 45°	Level of T6–7	14 × 17 in. lw	Entire chest. The right lung should be approximately twice the size of the left lung.
Right lateral decubitus	Horizontal beam	Level of T6–7	14 × 17 in. cw	Entire chest. An air–fluid level would be demonstrated in the right lung if fluid is present; a pneumothorax in the left lung would be demonstrated if present.

WORD SEARCH

```
S A M H Y C E S D C A Z A P K
I I P N E U M O N I A M R K X
S O T N F M E B J J H J A X G
O B B I E W O Y T T W E H F F
L Q R A T A A T S Q H Y M T U
U R O M H T N A H I P W T J H
C P N E U M O T H O R A X J S
R N C S I P I L X Z R U E S R
E C H Y Y C T I G T C A E C R
B E I H W K A U W I Q P X L H
U Y T P A K R S R D P O C T P
T Z I M A S I H I C C E C E T
I X S E R N P E R T U S S I S
U C Y A N O S I S P A X I G W
O D S L O Y A O X S H J U Y P
```

WORD LIST:

1. ASTHMA
2. APNEA
3. COPD
4. TUBERCULOSIS
5. BRONCHITIS
6. PLEURISY
7. EMPHYSEMA
8. PNEUMONIA
9. HYPOXIA
10. HEMOTHORAX
11. CYANOSIS
12. PERTUSSIS
13. ASPIRATION
14. EPIGLOTTIS
15. PNEUMOTHORAX

DISCUSSION OF ATYPICAL CASE STUDIES ◄

1. This case study involves the woman who is unable to stand for a CXR because she has had both legs amputated. It may be possible to perform this radiographic exam with the woman remaining in the wheelchair. If the chair is wide enough to accommodate a 14 × 17 in. cassette it can be slid down behind her for the AP. The lateral could be done if the arms of the wheelchair detach and the woman is able to move forward away from the chair back safely. If the CXR cannot be accomplished in this manner, she could be transferred onto a stretcher.

2. The patient who has a Swan–Ganz catheter in his femoral vein must remain in the supine or lateral position. The patient should be positioned on his right side to visualize the pleural effusion, which would look lighter than the lung tissue, and be on the down side of the radiograph.

3 ABDOMEN

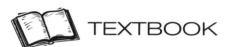 TEXTBOOK

Objectives

Following the completion of this chapter, the student will be able to:

1. Name and identify those structures contained within the abdominopelvic cavity, to include the digestive system, urinary system, adrenal glands, hepatobiliary system, spleen, and pancreas.
2. Describe the shape, relative position, and function of the diaphragm within the abdomen.
3. Differentiate between the four-quadrant and nine-region methods of localization of structures within the abdominopelvic cavity and identify structures normally located in each quadrant and/or region.
4. Identify those organs that are most affected by bodily habitus.
5. Define the terminology associated with the abdomen, to include anatomy, procedures, and pathology.
6. Describe the procedure for obtaining supine, prone, upright, and decubitus projections of the abdomen.
7. Describe the correct breathing instructions for radiography of the abdomen.
8. Identify the bony landmarks used for positioning the abdomen when taking supine, prone, upright, and decubitus projections.
9. List and describe the type and size of film holder, central ray location, and structures best demonstrated on supine, prone, upright, and decubitus projections of the abdomen.
10. Discuss the technical considerations needed for producing optimum radiographs of the abdomen.
11. Discuss how these technical considerations must be changed to accommodate the pediatric patient.
12. Identify those structures that should be visible, in reference to soft tissue differentiation, on a correctly exposed abdominal radiograph.
13. Practice the positioning for supine, prone, upright, and decubitus projections of the abdomen on another student or phantom.
14. Evaluate radiographs of the abdomen in terms of positioning, centering, image quality, and radiographic anatomy.
15. Differentiate between radiographs of the abdomen taken in the supine, prone, upright, and decubitus positions.
16. Discuss several critical considerations when performing bedside radiography of the abdomen.
17. Identify alternate methods of imaging various abdominal structures.

Chapter Outline

► SAMPLE 50-MINUTE LESSON

PREPARATION STEP   ESTIMATED TIME—10 MINUTES

A. Assemble teaching aids
   1. Overhead projector
   2. Overhead transparencies
      a. included in *Instructor's Resource Manual*
      b. trace drawings from *Applications Manual* on clear radiographic film
   3. Skeleton
   4. Anatomy model
   5. Radiographs
B. Introduce topic of positioning of the abdomen. Lecture will include Chapter Objectives 6 to 10.
C. Opening discussion
   1. At this point we will be learning how to perform abdomen radiographs when there is no exogenous contrast added. There are many subtle shades on an abdomen radiograph so technique is critical.
   2. The patients can be very ill. It is important to be aware of their physical status at all times.
   3. A grid should be used for all the abdomen radiographs that will be discussed. Male patients should be shielded; however, you will not be able to shield female patients. All the abdominal radiographs should be done on expiration. The right or left marker must be placed on the correct side so it obstructs as little of the abdomen as possible, and the patient identification area should always be placed down.

PRESENTATION STEP   ESTIMATED TIME—40 MINUTES

TEACHING OUTLINE	TEACHING AIDS & METHODS
I. Positioning of the Abdomen	
A. Supine AP Abdomen	
1. technical considerations	*AP abdomen radiograph*
a. 14 × 17 in. lengthwise film	
b. two crosswise if large patient	
c. SID—40 in.	
2. positioning	
a. patient supine on table	
3. central ray	
a. perpendicular to table	
b. center at iliac crests	
4. structures visualized	
a. renal shadows, psoas major muscles, transverse processes of the lumbar spine, inferior margin of the liver should be clearly visualized on a properly exposed abdominal radiograph	
b. *must include symphysis pubis*	
B. Upright AP Abdomen	
1. technical considerations	*Upright AP abdomen radiograph*
a. 14 × 17 in. lengthwise film	
b. two crosswise if large patient	
c. SID—40 in.	

2. positioning
   a. patient in erect position with back to upright table or wall unit
   b. patient may be seated on stool, stretcher, or bed
3. central ray
   a. parallel to floor
     (1) if patient is semierect do NOT angle tube
   b. center 2–3 in. above iliac crests
   c. center cassette to the central ray
   d. if specifically looking for free air may center *on* diaphragm
4. structures visualized
   a. should demonstrate renal shadows and psoas muscles
   b. air–fluid levels if present
   c. if free air present will be under right hemidiaphragm
   d. *must include diaphragm*

Demonstrate with clear glass of colored liquid

C. Left Lateral Decubitus Abdomen
  1. technical considerations
   a. 14 × 17 in. film
   b. SID—40 in.
  2. positioning
   a. patient in left lateral position
   b. elevate patient on decubitus board
   c. arms up and out of field
  3. central ray
   a. horizontal to center of cassette
   b. center 2–3 in. above iliac crests
  4. structures visualized
   a. should demonstrate diaphragm, renal shadows, and psoas muscles
   b. air–fluid levels if present
   c. free air if present will be between liver and diaphragm on the patient's right side
   d. *must include diaphragm*

Left lateral decubitus radiograph

D. Dorsal Decubitus Abdomen
  1. technical considerations
   a. 14 × 17 in. film
   b. SID—40 in.
  2. positioning
   a. patient in supine position
   b. elevate patient on decubitus board
  3. central ray
   a. horizontal to center of cassette
   b. center 2 in. above iliac crests, and 2 in. anterior to the midaxillary line of the patient
  4. structures visualized
   a. should demonstrate diaphragm, spine, and anterior margin of the abdomen air–fluid levels if present
   b. *must include diaphragm*

Dorsal decubitus radiograph

| APPLICATION STEP | ESTIMATED TIME—2 HOURS |

Study Assignment

A. Continue reading Chapter 3 in the text.
B. Be able to name all the anatomy studied in this chapter that is visualized on the abdominal radiographs.
C. Critique the abdominal radiographs for image quality and proper positioning.
D. Finish Chapter 3 in the *Applications Manual.*

| TESTING STEP |

Questions on this material will be included in exam given at end of Chapter 3.

► EXAM QUESTIONS

Matching

1. _____ Greater trochanter
2. _____ Iliac crest
3. _____ Symphysis pubis
4. _____ Ischial tuberosity
5. _____ Lumbar spine

A. column of bone located posterior in the abdominopelvic cavity
B. upper curved border of the ilium
C. large projection on the lateral femur
D. prominent projection of the pelvis located anteriorly
E. structure that is shaped like a shovel
F. bears weight when you sit down
G. anterior junction of the pubic bones

Multiple Choice

6. How is it possible to locate the stomach on a radiograph of the abdomen when the patient has NOT been given barium contrast to drink?
   A. the body of the stomach visualizes because it is surrounded by a layer of fat
   B. the pyloric sphincter is a dense structure that visualizes well
   C. the fundus of the stomach visualizes when it has an air bubble in it
   D. the stomach can be seen only when it is filled with barium

7. Name the parts of the colon in order starting with the ileocecal valve.
   A. cecum, ascending colon, splenic flexure, transverse colon, hepatic flexure, descending colon, sigmoid, rectum
   B. cecum, ascending colon, hepatic flexure, transverse colon, splenic flexure, descending colon, sigmoid, rectum
   C. cecum, descending colon, splenic flexure, transverse colon, hepatic flexure, ascending colon, sigmoid, rectum
   D. ascending colon, splenic flexure, transverse colon, descending colon, hepatic flexure, rectum, cecum, sigmoid

8. Which of the following positions demonstrates free air in the abdomen?
   1. supine
   2. upright

3. left lateral decubitus

    A. 1 only

    B. 1 and 2 only

    C. 2 and 3 only

    D. 1, 2, and 3

9. For which type of radiograph is the centering point the iliac crest?

    A. upright AP abdomen

    B. supine AP abdomen

    C. left lateral decubitus abdomen

    D. dorsal decubitus abdomen

10. What structure must be included on a supine AP radiograph of the abdomen?

    A. diaphragm

    B. ischial tuberosity

    C. symphysis pubis

    D. base of the lungs

11. What structure must be included on a upright AP radiograph of the abdomen?

    A. diaphragm

    B. symphysis pubis

    C. greater tuberosity

    D. ischial tuberosity

12. You are doing a left lateral decubitus of the abdomen on a very large patient. The exam is being done portably and you only have one film. Which is the most important side of the patient to visualize for free air?

    A. the patient's left side

    B. the patient's right side

13. How is it possible to visualize the renal shadow on an abdominal film taken before contrast is injected?

    A. the kidneys are surrounded by air

    B. the kidneys are located below the adrenal glands, which are highly visible on an abdominal radiograph

    C. the kidneys are composed of calcium, which makes them easy to visualize

    D. the kidneys are surrounded by an adipose capsule, which is often discernible on an abdomen radiograph

14. Bile is produced in the _____ and stored and concentrated in the _____ .

    A. liver, gallbladder

    B. gallbladder, liver

    C. kidneys, gallbladder

    D. gallbladder, biliary ducts

15. The muscles that run at an oblique angle in the abdomen and originate at the bodies and transverse processes of T-12 through L-5 are named the:

    A. costophrenic muscles

    B. diaphragm

    C. vertebral muscles

    D. psoas muscles

Answer Key

1. C	4. F	7. B	10. C	13. D
2. B	5. A	8. C	11. A	14. A
3. G	6. C	9. B	12. B	15. D

 APPLICATIONS MANUAL

▶ DRAWINGS

Coloring the abdomen drawings may be a little trickier than the chest, but the students should be able to color the bony anatomy, kidneys, and parts of the colon, each a different color. You might ask them to draw in what free air would look like on the Left Lateral Decubitus drawing.

▶ ANSWER KEY FOR STUDY QUESTIONS

1. Diaphragm
2. Peritoneum
3. Mesentery and omentum
4. _____

right hypochondriac	epigastric	left hypochondriac
right lumbar	umbilicus	left lumbar
right iliac	hypogastric	left iliac

5. Left hypochondriac
6. _____

right upper quadrant	left upper quadrant
right lower quadrant	left lower quadrant

7. Right lower quadrant
8. Right upper quadrant
9. It affects the size, shape, and relative position of the internal organs, particularly the stomach and gallbladder.
10. 12
11. It is located posteriorly on the midline of the body.
12. Lumbar spine
13. Sacrum
14. Coccyx

15. Spinous processes
16. Between the bodies of the vertebrae
17. Ala
18. The disk space between the 4th and 5th lumbar vertebrae
19. Anterior superior iliac spine (ASIS)
20. Symphysis pubis
21. Ischial tuberosity
22. Obturator
23. The urinary bladder is located directly posterior to the symphysis pubis.
24. Greater trochanter
25. A hemidiaphragm is that portion of the diaphragm under the right or the left lung.
26. Psoas major
27. It is the continuous hollow tube of the digestive system.
28. The psoas major muscles are located laterally to the vertebral column and attach to the bodies and transverse processes of the 12th thoracic through 5th lumbar vertebrae.
29. Pharynx; anus
30. The 10th thoracic vertebra
31. Cardiac antrum; less than 1 in. (1–2 cm)
32. The stomach spans the epigastric, umbilical, and left hypochondriac regions of the abdomen.
33. The stomach is generally J-shaped.
34. Rugae
35. Pyloric orifice
36. Fundus, body, and pyloric antrum
37. In the fundus of the stomach
38. Duodenum, jejunum, and ileum
39. 20 ft (6 m)
40. Duodenum
41. Ileum
42. Left upper and left lower quadrants
43. Right lower quadrant
44. The large intestine is located around the periphery of the abdominopelvic cavity, while the small intestine generally occupies a more central location.
45. Cecum
46. Hepatic flexure
47. Sigmoid colon
48. Right
49. Haustra are sacs or pouches formed along the length of the large intestine.
50. Cecum
51. By the size, shape, and location of the gas. The large intestine is larger in diameter, has haustra, and is located around the periphery of the abdomen, while the small intestine is generally smaller in diameter, looks like stacked coins or a coiled wire, and is more centrally located.
52. The urinary system functions to remove waste and excess water from the body.
53. Because they are located behind the peritoneum
54. The presence of the adipose (fatty) capsule surrounding the kidneys
55. The right kidney is lower due to the presence of the liver above it.
56. Ureters
57. The urinary bladder is located posteriorly to the symphysis pubis and under the peritoneum (infraperitoneal).
58. The adrenal (suprarenal) glands
59. Right
60. Gallbladder
61. Common bile duct
62. Liver
63. Cystic duct

64. The female reproductive organs are located within the abdominopelvic cavity. If they were covered by lead shielding, other important anatomy may be obscured.
65. The uterus is situated anterior to the rectum and posterosuperior to the urinary bladder.
66. Ovaries
67. Tubal ligation
68. Hysterectomy
69. Uterine (fallopian) tubes (oviducts)
70. Testes
71. Yes; lead shielding can usually be applied without compromising other important anatomy because the male reproductive organs are located primarily below the symphysis pubis.
72. Prostate gland
73. Pancreas
74. The spleen is located between the stomach and left kidney.
75. Aorta
76. Inferior vena cava (IVC)
77. Spleen
78. Transposition or situs inversus
79. Laparoscopy
80. The elastic on the underpants may create unwanted artifacts and areas of inconsistent density on the radiograph.
81. To allow air in the abdomen to rise and fluid to settle
82. It is a recumbent AP or PA projection of the abdomen which includes the kidneys, ureters, and urinary bladder.
83. The pillow or sponge acts as a support for the knees and relieves stress on the lower back.
84. The iliac crest
85. Since the urinary bladder lies posteriorly to the symphysis pubis, the radiographer can palpate either the greater trochanters of the femurs, which are 1½ in above the symphysis pubis, or the ischial tuberosities, which are 1½ in below the symphysis pubis.
86. Upright abdomen, left lateral decubitus abdomen, and PA upright chest
87. Take the upright projection first. Since the patient was already sitting erect in the wheelchair, any fluid should have settled and air risen, allowing air–fluid levels to be demonstrated satisfactorily.
88. It is a series of radiographs of the abdomen, to include AP or PA recumbent, upright, and/or left lateral decubitus projections. Some departmental routines also require an upright PA projection of the chest.
89. Approximately 2–3 in. above the iliac crests
90. The right and left ilia should appear symmetrical; the ribs should appear symmetrical bilaterally; and the bodies of the lumbar vertebrae should appear boxlike with the spinous processes in a straight line.
91. The abdominal aorta is located posteriorly in the abdomen. When calcified, it is demonstrated just anterior to the lumbar vertebrae.
92. 70–80 kVp
93. Hysterosalpingogram; either water-soluble or oily iodinated
94. When a person lies on his/her left side, the liver drops slightly, creating a space between it and the diaphragm referred to as the subphrenic space. Any free air in the abdomen would be visible in the subphrenic space.
95. True
96. False; radiographs of the abdomen should be taken on exhalation so that the abdominal organs are not displaced inferiorly.
97. True
98. True
99. True

100.

Projection	CR Angle/ Angle of Part	Centering Point	Film Size	Structures Seen
PA recumbent abdomen	CR = perpendicular part = 0°	Iliac crests	14 × 17 in. lw	Renal shadows, psoas major muscles, pubic symphysis, inferior margin of the liver, lumbosacral spine
AP upright abdomen	CR = horizontal part = 0°	Approx. 2–3 in. above iliac crest	14 × 17 in. lw	Diaphragm, air–fluid levels within the bowel, renal shadows, psoas major muscles, inferior margin of liver
Left lateral decubitus abdomen	CR = horizontal part = 0°	Approx. 2–3 in. above iliac crest	14 × 17 in. lw with patient's body	Diaphragm, air–fluid levels within the bowel

▶ ANSWER KEY FOR CROSSWORD PUZZLE

```
 1             2
 I  N  C  O    N  T  I  N  E  N  C  E
 N             A                    3                 4
 G          5  U  B  A  L  L  I  G  A  T  I  O  N     A
 U          5  T                    H                 S
 I          S                       A                 C
 N       6  I  L  E  U  S     7  P  E  R  I  S  T  A  L  S  I  S
 A          A                       A                 T
 A                                  L                 E
 8  9    10                                           S
 L  A  P  A  R  O  S  C  O  P  Y
    P     N                   11
 12 P  N  E  U  M  O  P  E  R  C  T  O  N  E  U  M
    E     U                   I
    N     R        13         N                    14
    D     Y        E          S                    V
    I     S        M          S                    O
    C     M     15 E  A  U  N  D  I  C  E          L
    I           J  S          P                    V
    I              I       16 C  A  L  C  17 U  L  U  S
 18 S  T  E  N  O  S  I  S     A        L
    I                         T        C
 19 H  Y  S  T  E  R  E  C  T  O  M  Y  E
                              O        R
                              N
```

ACROSS

1. incontinence
5. tubal ligation
6. ileus
7. peristalsis
8. laparoscopy
12. pneumoperitoneum
15. jaundice
16. calculus
18. stenosis
19. hysterectomy

DOWN

1. inguinal
2. nausea
3. hiatal
4. ascites
9. appendicitis
10. aneurysm
11. constipation
13. emesis
14. volvulus
17. ulcer

1. An 11 × 14 in. supine radiograph could be performed to include the area from the mouth to anus of the 3-year-old child who swallowed a quarter, as long as the child is not experiencing breathing difficulties. An abdomen technique would visualize the quarter wherever it has lodged. The centering point would be in the middle of the film at approximately the diaphragm. A lateral neck would demonstrate whether the quarter was lodged in the trachea (anterior neck) or esophagus (posterior neck).

2. This case study describes a scene in which an upright and supine abdomen radiograph has been ordered on a woman in obvious pain who is vomiting. An upright abdomen radiograph could be performed with the patient on the table if it tilts into an upright position. As the upright has been ordered to visualize free air, the central ray should be centered on the diaphragm. If the patient is not able to tolerate being in the upright position, a left lateral decubitus would also visualize free air.

4 INTRODUCTION TO THE MUSCULOSKELETAL SYSTEM

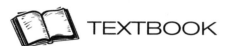 TEXTBOOK

Objectives

Following the completion of this chapter, the student will be able to:

1. List four functions of the skeletal system.
2. Define terminology of the musculoskeletal system, to include anatomy, procedures, and pathology related to bones, joints, and muscles.
3. Identify the two divisions of the skeleton and list the number of bones in each division.
4. Differentiate between the classifications of bones according to shape and give examples of each.
5. Describe the basic anatomical structure of bone.
6. Identify and describe the various features, including markings, found on the surfaces of bones.
7. Discuss the process of bone development and growth.
8. List and describe the three main classifications of joints and give examples of each.
9. Identify several causes of skeletal disorders.
10. Distinguish between various types of fractures.
11. Describe the fracture process, to include physical signs of fracture and the healing process.
12. Discuss the three classifications of muscles.
13. Differentiate between muscles, ligaments, and tendons.
14. Describe four functions of muscles.
15. Differentiate between the four functional characteristics of skeletal muscles.
16. Discuss the technical and equipment considerations involved in producing optimum radiographs of the skeletal system.
17. Discuss how the technical and equipment factors must be modified to accommodate pediatric and geriatric patients.
18. Explain the rationale for taking a minimum of two projections at 90° from each other when radiographing the skeletal system.
19. Discuss the need for an additional (oblique) projection when radiographing a joint.
20. Describe the procedural and technical modifications to be considered when performing a radiographic exam of an extremity in a cast or splint.
21. Describe the appropriate procedure for imaging the skeletal system at the patient's bedside.
22. Discuss the need for adjusting technical factors for various pathologic conditions of the skeletal system.
23. Identify alternative methods of imaging bones and articulations.

Chapter Outline

I. SKELETAL ANATOMY
   A. Functions
      1. support
      2. protection
      3. movement
      4. storage
      5. hematopoiesis
   B. Classification
      1. long
      2. short
      3. flat
      4. irregular
      5. sesamoid
      6. wormian
   C. Bone Growth and Development
      1. intramembranous ossification
      2. endochondral ossification
   D. Bone Physiology
   E. Bone Markings
   F. Bony Pathologies

II. ARTHROLOGY
   A. Synarthrosis/Fibrous
   B. Amphiarthrosis/Cartilaginous/Fibrous
   C. Diathrosis/Synovial
      1. ball and socket
      2. condyloid
      3. saddle
      4. hinge
      5. pivot
      6. gliding

III. MUSCULAR ANATOMY
   A. Classification
      1. skeletal
      2. visceral
      3. cardiac
   B. Function
      1. movement
      2. posture
      3. support
      4. heat
   C. Attachment
      1. origin
      2. insertion
   D. Associated Structures
      1. tendon
      2. ligament

E. Naming System
1. shape
2. size
3. sections
4. location
5. direction of fibers
6. action
7. origin/insertion

IV. RELATED TERMINOLOGY

V. PROCEDURAL CONSIDERATIONS
A. Patient Preparations
B. Positioning Considerations
C. Breathing Instructions
D. Exposure Factors
E. Equipment Considerations
F. Orthopedic Cast Radiography
G. Pediatric and Geriatric Patients
H. Special Skeletal Procedures
1. metastatic bone survey/bone survey
2. dialysis survey
3. bone age studies
4. child abuse diagnosis series
I. Bedside Radiography
J. Alternate Imaging Methods
1. tomography
2. computed tomography
3. arthrography
4. magnetic resonance imaging
5. nuclear medicine
6. myelography
7. diskography

VI. SUMMARY

VII. CRITICAL THINKING & APPLICATION QUESTIONS

◄ SAMPLE 50-MINUTE LESSON

| PREPARATION STEP | ESTIMATED TIME—10 MINUTES |

A. Assemble teaching aids
1. Overhead projector
2. Overhead transparencies
a. included in *Instructor's Resource Manual*
3. Skeleton
4. Radiographs
B. Lecture in a continuation of Chapter 4 and will cover Chapter Objectives 8 to 11.

C. Opening discussion
   1. Extremely important information is contained in this chapter
   2. You must learn the information well as it forms the basic structure needed to learn all the anatomy, positioning, and pathology of the musculoskeletal system.

PRESENTATION STEP   ESTIMATED TIME—40 MINUTES

TEACHING OUTLINE	TEACHING AIDS & METHODS
I. Arthrology	
A. Study of joints/articulations	*Arthrology transparency*
B. Almost every bone in the body articulates with at least one other bone to form a joint	
C. Classified according to function and structure	
D. Functional classification	
1. synarthrosis	
a. immovable	
2. amphiarthrosis	
a. slightly movable	
3. diarthrosis	
a. freely movable	
E. Structural classification	*Refer to transparency for specific*
1. fibrous	*details and exceptions*
a. suture	
b. synchondrosis	
c. synostosis	
d. gomphosis	
2. cartilaginous	
a. symphysis	
b. syndesmosis*	**Explain that this type of joint is*
3. synovial	*actually fibrous but permits slight*
a. ball and socket	*movement*
b. condyloid	
c. saddle	
d. hinge	
e. pivot	
f. gliding	
II. Skeletal Disorders	
A. Conditions that can interrupt normal homeostasis and cause skeletal disorders	
1. congenital defects	
a. talipes equinovarus (clubfoot)	
(1) foot turns downward and inward	
2. hormone imbalance	
a. osteoporosis	
(1) strongly related to lack of estrogen after menopause	
3. malnutrition	
a. osteomalacia / rickets	
(1) vitamin D deficiency	
4. degenerative diseases	
a. Paget's disease	

        5. inflammatory diseases
           a. osteomyelitis
        6. injuries
           a. fractures
   III. Fractures
        A. Classifications   *Transparency of fracture types*
           1. outward appearance
              a. closed vs. open
           2. mechanics of injury   *Radiographic fracture examples*
              a. spiral
           3. site / location
              a. Colles' fracture of the radius
           4. usually more than one criteria will apply
        B. Signs radiographer should be aware of
           1. abnormal movement or motion of part
           2. differences in shape and length
              between sides
           3. obvious deformities
              a. large bump
              b. misalignment
           4. open wound over bone
           5. swelling
           6. discoloration
           7. pain or tenderness
        C. Healing process
           1. fracture hematoma
           2. internal and external callus forms
           3. cartilage of external callus replaced by bone
           4. spongy bone replaced by compact bone

APPLICATION STEP   ESTIMATED TIME—2 HOURS

Study Assignment

A. Continue reading Chapter 4 in the text.
B. Continue Chapter 4 in the *Applications Manual.*
C. Study the information contained in this chapter thoroughly. It is very important information that
   will help you learn the subsequent chapters, which deal with anatomy and positioning of the skeletal system.

TESTING STEP

Questions on this material will be included in exam given at end of Chapter 4.

◄ EXAM QUESTIONS

Matching

1. _____ Closed fracture   A. bone fractures across long axis

2. _____ Compound fracture   B. bone broken into small fragments

3. _____ Communited fracture   C. occurs in vertebrae when subjected to extreme stress

4. _____ Avulsion fracture

5. _____ Greenstick fracture

D. fracture projects through skin

E. one side of shaft is broken, other side is bent

F. skin around fracture is not broken

G. chip of bone pulled away by tearing of ligament attachment

Multiple Choice

6. The rapid form of bone growth that takes place primarily in flat bones such as the calvarium is termed:
   A. endochondral ossification
   B. intramembranous ossification
   C. epiphyseal ossification
   D. metaphysis ossification

7. The name of the disease that results from a deficiency of vitamin D in children is:
   A. osteopenia
   B. osteomalacia
   C. rickets
   D. Paget's

8. The joint between the roots of the teeth and the bony socket of the maxillae and mandible bones is termed:
   A. symphysis
   B. syndesmosis
   C. synchrondrosis
   D. gomphosis

9. A sac of synovial fluid that is positioned between tissues around a joint is called a
   A. synovial membrane
   B. bursa
   C. joint capsule
   D. condyle

10. Which type of articulation allows movement in a single plane in the form of flexion and extension?
    A. saddle
    B. pivot
    C. hinge
    D. gliding

11. Which type of articulation allows the most movement?
    A. ball and socket
    B. condyloid
    C. saddle
    D. pivot

12. A band of white fibrous connective tissue that connects a muscle to a bone is called a
    A. ligament
    B. tendon
    C. menisci
    D. muscle attachment

Answer Key

1. F	4. G	7. C	10. C
2. D	5. E	8. D	11. A
3. B	6. B	9. B	12. B

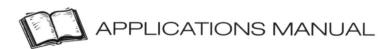

APPLICATIONS MANUAL

► ANSWER KEY FOR STUDY QUESTIONS

1. The scientific study of bones
2. 206
3. A. support
   B. protection
   C. movement
   D. storage
   E. hematopoiesis
4. Compact and cancellous
5. 20%
6. Cancellous
7. In the haversian canals
8. Trabeculae
9. Periosteum
10. Diaphysis
11. Medullary; bone marrow
12. Cortical bone is another name for compact bone because it forms the cortex or outer shell of the bone.
13. It lines the medullary cavity.
14. The carpals are short bones.
15. Nutrient foramen
16. Sesamoid bones
17. They are sutural bones that develop between the joints of the cranial bones.
18. Axial and appendicular
19. Any of the following: sternum, ilium, bones of the skull cap
20. Ossification
21. It is the area of growth at the end of the diaphysis, where the epiphyseal plate is located.
22. Intramembranous ossification
23. The metaphyses (distal ends of diaphysis)
24. The presence of epiphyseal plates at the distal end of the femur and proximal tibia and fibula. Since the epiphyses of these bones have not fused to the diaphyses, growth is still taking place.
25. Epiphyses
26. There are four steps to the remodeling process: (1) development of a hematoma, (2) callus formation, (3) replacement of the callus with spongy bone, and (4) replacement of spongy bone with compact bone.
27. Osteoclasts
28. Osteocytes
29. Callus appears as a white haziness around the fracture site.
30. A. 11
    B. 5
    C. 7
    D. 2

E. 14

F. 1

G. 12

H. 9

I. 6

J. 10

31. Osteomyelitis

32. Fracture

33. Osteoporosis

34. A. abnormal movement of the body part

B. difference in length and shape of corresponding bones on the two sides of the patient's body

C. obvious deformities, such as a large bump or misalignment of articulating bones

D. an open wound over the bone

E. swelling or the soft tissue around the injury

F. discoloration (blanching or redness) of the skin at the site of the injury

G. pain or tenderness in response to gentle pressure at the site of the injury

35. Avulsion

36. Open/compound

37. Torus

38. Spiral

39. Comminuted

40. An articulation is a joint formed by the juncture of two or more bones.

41. Synarthrosis, amphiarthrosis, and diarthrosis

42. Sutures

43. Symphysis

44. Gomphoses; synarthrodial

45. A syndesmosis is an amphiarthrodial joint that is fibrous in structure, allowing slight movement. The distal tibiofibular joint is an example.

46. Initially, it is a synchondrosis because cartilage is present. As the child matures, the epiphysis and diaphysis eventually fuse together into a completely immovable joint called a synostosis.

47. A diarthrodial joint has a joint capsule and the articular surfaces of the bones are covered with hyaline cartilage. A synarthrodial joint has no joint capsule and the bones are joined by fibrous connective tissue.

48. Structural classification—synovial; functional classification—diarthrodial with ball and socket movement

49. It is found in diarthrodial joints where it provides nourishment to the articular cartilage and lubricates it to reduce friction during movement.

50. Menisci

51. Ball and socket, condyloid, saddle, pivot, hinge, and gliding

52. Saddle joint; either the 1st metacarpophalangeal or 1st carpometacarpal joint

53. Pivot

54. Muscle

55. Skeletal, visceral, and cardiac

56. Movement, posture, support, and heat

57. Ligament

58. Because they can be controlled at command, unlike visceral and cardiac muscles

59. Visceral

60. Sphincter

61. They are both points of attachment of the muscle. The origin is the more fixed attachment at the proximal end and the insertion is the more movable attachment at the distal end of the muscle.

62. Strain

63. At least two projections 90° from each other

64. Precisely where the bruise is located, the appearance (color, etc) of the bruise, how the injury occurred, when the injury occurred, and any complaint of pain, discomfort, etc, by the patient.

65. To demonstrate all surfaces of the joint
66. Decrease
67. D
68. A
69. A
70. D
71. D
72. It would improve visualization of detail, particularly of the small carpal bones.
73. They are taken to assess the alignment and position of the fractured bone after the physician has reduced the fracture (manipulated the part).
74. If the fiberglass cast is dry, no change in technique should be needed. If the cast is still wet, the kVp may be increased slightly (0–4 kVp) depending upon the degree of wetness.
75. The detail in the cast detracts from the bony anatomy and fine detail is not needed for cast radiography, as it is usually performed to check alignment of bones and not to detect small fractures. In addition, the use of a faster speed film/screen system would minimize the patient's dose for this exam.
76. Elderly patients often have a lack of muscle tone and decreased mineralization of the bones. The use of higher kVp overpenetrates the part.
77. A skeletal survey is commonly performed to evaluate the demineralization of bones, which can occur in patients with chronic renal disease.
78. Arthrography
79. A Bone Age Study is performed to determine whether a child's growth is accelerated or delayed for his/her chronologic age. The extremities (usually the hand and wrist) are radiographed and then compared to a chart depicting the standards for each age and sex.

WORD SEARCH

```
S  I  D  L  L  G  E  R  U  T  U  S  M  G  J
I  G  I  S  Y  E  I  R  G  D  J  R  N  X  I
S  O  F  C  Y  R  A  L  U  G  E  R  R  I  J
E  D  G  I  H  G  J  L  M  T  N  D  N  C  A
I  N  H  D  J  U  O  Q  U  O  C  G  Q  R  I
O  S  T  E  O  M  A  L  A  C  I  A  T  Z  V
P  F  F  P  V  K  P  Q  O  L  E  H  R  L  I
O  L  L  O  N  G  S  K  U  Y  R  B  Q  F  M
T  S  S  H  G  R  V  X  S  O  M  G  A  U  K
A  A  R  T  H  R  A  L  G  I  A  T  S  R  L
M  F  T  R  R  T  Y  R  J  P  Z  C  D  K  T
E  C  F  O  I  A  A  N  K  Y  L  O  S  I  S
H  E  Q  O  B  M  I  B  M  E  N  B  E  Q  K
F  T  N  A  J  S  Z  N  S  F  D  M  D  X  M
```

WORD LIST

1. ANKYLOSIS
2. ARTHRALGIA
3. ARTHROGRAM
4. FRACTURE
5. HEMATOPOIESIS
6. IRREGULAR
7. LONG
8. LUXATION
9. MUSCLES
10. MYOLOGY
11. ORTHOPEDICS
12. OSTEOMALACIA
13. STRAIN
14. SUTURE
15. TRABECULAE

UPPER LIMB (EXTREMITY) 5

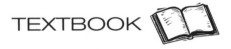

TEXTBOOK

Objectives

Following the completion of this chapter, the student will be able to:

1. Given diagrams, radiographs, or dry bones, name and describe the bones of the upper limb, to include the hand, wrist, forearm, and humerus.
2. Identify any surface markings found on the bones of the upper limb.
3. List any additional names for the bones or structures of the upper limb, specifically the carpal bones.
4. Classify the articulations in the upper limb and identify their type of movement.
5. List and describe the basic projections of the upper limb, to include preferred type and size of image receptor, central ray location, and structures best visualized.
6. Describe the positioning steps for taking supplemental projections of the upper limb due to trauma, pain, etc.
7. Describe equipment considerations and exposure factors relative to radiography of the upper limb.
8. Practice positioning the basic projections of the upper limb on another student or phantom.
9. State the criteria used to determine positioning accuracy on radiographs of the upper limb.
10. Evaluate radiographs of the upper limb in terms of positioning, centering, image quality, radiographic anatomy, and pathology.
11. Define terminology associated with the upper limb, to include anatomy, procedures, and pathology.

Chapter Outline

I. ANATOMY OF THE UPPER LIMB
   A. Hand and Wrist
      1. phalanges
      2. metacarpals
      3. carpals
   B. Forearm
      1. radius
      2. ulna
   C. Upper Arm
   D. Humerus

II. ARTHROLOGY OF THE UPPER LIMB
   A. Interphalangeal Joints
   B. First Metacarpophalangeal Joint
   C. Second Through Fifth Metacarpophalangeal Joints
   D. First Carpometacarpal Joint
   E. Second Through Fifth Carpometacarpal Joints
   F. Intercarpal
   G. Radiocarpal
   H. Distal Radioulnar
   I. Proximal Radioulnar
   J. Elbow
   K. Shoulder

III. PROCEDURAL CONSIDERATIONS
   A. Patient Preparations
   B. Positioning Considerations
   C. Exposure Factors
   D. Equipment Considerations

IV. RADIOGRAPHIC POSITIONING OF THE UPPER LIMB
   A. Fingers (2nd–5th Digits): PA, Oblique, Lateral
      1. technical considerations
      2. shielding
      3. patient positioning
      4. part positioning
      5. central ray
      6. image evaluation
      7. critical anatomy
   B. Thumb (1st Digit): AP, Oblique, Lateral
      1. technical considerations
      2. shielding
      3. patient positioning
      4. part positioning
      5. central ray
      6. image evaluation
      7. critical anatomy
   C. Hand: PA, Oblique, Lateral
      1. technical considerations
      2. shielding
      3. patient positioning
      4. part positioning
      5. central ray
      6. image evaluation
      7. critical anatomy
   D. Wrist: PA, PA Oblique, AP Oblique, Lateral, PA in Radial Flexion, Tangential Carpal Canal
      1. technical considerations
      2. shielding
      3. patient positioning
      4. part positioning

      5. central ray

      6. image evaluation

      7. critical anatomy

  E. Forearm: AP, Lateral

      1. technical considerations

      2. shielding

      3. patient positioning

      4. part positioning

      5. central ray

      6. image evaluation

      7. critical anatomy

  F. Elbow: AP, AP in Partial Flexion, Medial Oblique, External Oblique, Lateral, Axial Lateral

      1. technical considerations

      2. shielding

      3. patient positioning

      4. part positioning

      5. central ray

      6. image evaluation

      7. critical anatomy

  G. Humerus: AP, Lateral, AP Neutral Position, Transthoracic Lateral

      1. technical considerations

      2. shielding

      3. patient positioning

      4. part positioning

      5. central ray

      6. image evaluation

      7. critical anatomy

 V. SUMMARY

 VI. CRITICAL THINKING & APPLICATION QUESTIONS

VII. FILM CRITIQUE

SAMPLE 50-MINUTE LESSON ◄

PREPARATION STEP   ESTIMATED TIME—10 MINUTES

A. Assemble teaching aids

  1. Overhead projector

  2. Overhead transparencies

    a. included in *Instructor's Resource Manual*

    b. trace drawings from *Applications Manual* on clear radiographic film

  3. Skeleton

  4. Radiographs

B. Introduce topic of anatomy of the upper limb. Lecture will include Chapter Objectives 1, 2, and 3.

C. Opening discussion

  1. Bony anatomy is easier to discern on a radiograph than soft tissue. Why?

  2. This chapter begins our tour through the bony anatomy of the body.

  3. You must not only learn the anatomy and positioning well, but must be able to visualize what anatomy is seen in each position learned. This is the purpose of the drawings in the workbook.

4. When terms *lateral* and *medial* are used in regard to the upper extremity, this is always done in relationship to the anatomic position.
5. This lecture will cover the specific anatomy of the hand, wrist, and forearm.

PRESENTATION STEP   ESTIMATED TIME—40 MINUTES

TEACHING OUTLINE	TEACHING AIDS & METHODS
I. Anatomy of the Upper Limb	*Show anatomy on skeleton*
A. Hand and Wrist	
1. digit 1 on lateral side	
2. digit 5 on medial side	
3. phalanges	
a. head—rounded distal end	*Hand and wrist transparency*
(1) ungulate process or tuft	
b. shaft	
c. base—flattened proximal end	*Hand and wrist radiographs*
d. thumb has two	
(1) distal and proximal	
e. digits 2 through 5 have three	
(1) distal, middle, and proximal	
4. metacarpals	
a. form palm of hand	
b. *meta* means beyond	
(1) metacarpal = beyond the carpals	
c. 1st metacarpal on lateral side	
d. 5th metacarpal on medial side	
e. head—rounded distal end	
f. shaft	
g. base flattened proximal end	
5. carpals	*Mnemonic for carpal bones transparency*
a. proximal row starting on lateral side	
(1) scaphoid/navicular	*Steve*
(a) boat-shaped	
(b) most commonly fractured carpal	
(2) lunate/semilunar	*Left*
(a) crescent-shaped	
(3) triquetrum/triangular/triquetral	*The*
(a) triangular-shaped	
(4) pisiform	*Party*
(a) pea-shaped	
(b) smallest carpal	
b. distal row starting on lateral side	
(1) trapezium/greater multangular	*To*
(a) four-sided bone	
(b) articulated with first metacarpal	
(2) trapezoid/lesser multangular	*Take*
(a) smaller four-sided bone	
(3) capitate/os magnum	*Carol*
(a) largest carpal	
(b) head-shaped	
(4) hamate/unciform	*Home*
(a) hook-shaped	
(i) hamular process	

B. Forearm
    1. radius   *Forearm transparency*
        a. lateral side of forearm
        b. base—distal end
            (1) broadest part   *Forearm radiographs*
            (2) concave surface articulates with scaphoid
            and lunate
            (3) styloid process
                (a) pointed conical process on lateral
                     aspect of base
        c. ulnar notch   Explanation: *Depression named for*
            (1) head of ulna fits in   *bone that fits in it*
        d. shaft/diaphysis
        e. head—proximal end
            (1) disk-shaped
            (2) fits into radial notch of ulna
        f. neck
            (1) constricted area
            (2) distal to head
        g. radial tuberosity   *Projection named for bone it is*
            (1) projection on anteromedial   *located on*
            aspect of radius
            (2) distal to neck
    2. ulna
        a. head—distal end
            (1) fits into ulnar notch of radius
            (2) styloid process
                (a) pointed process on medial side of head
        b. shaft/diaphysis
        c. olecranon process
            (1) pointed tip of elbow
        d. coronoid process
            (1) smaller beaklike process
            (2) anterior and inferior to olecranon
        e. radial notch
            (1) lateral side of coronoid
            (2) head of radius articulates
        f. trochlear/semilunar notch
            (1) articulates with trochlea of humerus

APPLICATION STEP   ESTIMATED TIME—3 HOURS

Study Assignment

A. Read Chapter 5 in the text.
B. Find all the anatomy discussed on the skeleton.
C. Find all the anatomy discussed on the radiographs of the upper arm.
D. Begin Chapter 5 in the *Applications Manual.*
E. Compare the positioning drawings in the *Applications Manual* to a corresponding radiograph.
F. Critique radiographs for image quality and proper positioning. Be sure you can locate the
   anatomic parts listed on the drawing worksheets on each of the radiographs.

TESTING STEP

Questions on this material will be included in exam given at end of this chapter.

▶ EXAM QUESTIONS

Multiple Choice

1. The lateral radiograph of the wrist shows two carpals slightly anterior. Which ones are they?
   A. pisiform and trapezium
   B. hamate and scaphoid
   C. capitate and lunate
   D. lunate and scaphoid

2. How would you describe the location of the head of the ulna on an AP radiograph?
   A. at the distal end and on the medial side of the arm
   B. at the distal end and on the lateral side of the arm
   C. at the proximal end and on the medial side of the arm
   D. at the proximal end and on the lateral side of the arm

3. Which of the following positions/projections would best demonstrate the pisiform free of superimposition?
   A. ulnar flexion
   B. radial flexion
   C. PA oblique
   D. AP oblique

4. Which of the following positions/projections would demonstrate forward or backward displacement of a fractured metacarpal?
   A. PA hand
   B. oblique hand
   C. lateral hand
   D. ulnar flexion

5. How should the patient be positioned to obtain an optimal lateral wrist?
   A. the elbow should be flexed at a 90° angle
   B. the elbow is extended and the radius and ulna are superimposed
   C. the elbow is hyperflexed
   D. the position of the elbow is unimportant when doing a lateral wrist radiograph

6. How should the hand be positioned to avoid superimposition of the proximal radius and ulna when doing a forearm radiograph?
   A. pronated
   B. supinated
   C. abducted
   D. adducted

7. What is the relationship of the surgical neck to the anatomical neck of the humerus?
   A. the surgical neck is distal to the anatomical neck
   B. the surgical neck is proximal to the anatomical neck

C. the surgical neck is just distal to the humeral head

D. the surgical neck is between the tubercles

8. Your radiograph visualizes the humeral epicondyles parallel to the film and includes the shoulder and elbow. What projection/position are you looking at?

A. AP humerus

B. lateral humerus

C. transthoracic humerus

D. view done to visualize the humerus

9. The patient is supine on the table. The grid cassette is against her left shoulder and you are using a cross-table beam. You are centered to the right armpit and the right arm is over the patient's head. What radiograph are you doing?

A. transthoracic humerus (left)

B. transthoracic humerus (right)

C. view done to visualize the humerus (left)

D. lateral humerus (right)

10. What is the main structure visualized when the central ray is angled 45° toward the shoulder through the humeral epicondyles and the patient's elbow is flexed 90°?

A. coronoid process

B. coronoid fossa

C. radial head

D. medial epicondyle

11. What structure is located between the olecranon process and the coronoid process on the ulna?

A. radial neck

B. styloid process of the ulna

C. trochlear notch

D. radial tuberosity

12. Which part of the ulna articulates with the radial head at the proximal radioulnar articulation?

A. capitulum

B. trochlea

C. radial tuberosity

D. radial notch

13. What structure on the humerus articulates with the most proximal portion of the ulna when the arm is extended?

A. coronoid fossa

B. olecranon fossa

C. trochlear notch

D. radial notch

14. Which radiograph primarily visualizes the olecranon process, trochlear notch, and radial tuberosity in profile?

A. AP elbow

B. medial oblique elbow

C. lateral oblique elbow

D. lateral elbow

15. Which radiograph is done to visualize the coronoid process?
   A. AP elbow
   B. medial oblique elbow
   C. lateral oblique elbow
   D. lateral elbow

ANSWER KEY

1. A	4. C	7. A	10. C	13. B
2. A	5. A	8. A	11. C	14. D
3. D	6. B	9. A	12. D	15. B

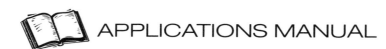 APPLICATIONS MANUAL

▶ DRAWINGS

Each type of bone should be colored a different color (ie, metacarpals). The carpals should be colored the same color on the hand drawings and labeled collectively. Each carpal should be colored a different color on the wrist drawings and labeled individually. The right and left markers are placed on the lateral side of the part. This is a common protocol, although many sites prefer to place the marker on the medial side on hand and wrist radiographs.

▶ ANSWER KEY FOR STUDY QUESTIONS

1. 14; digits
2. It is the roughened clump of bony tissue seen at the anterior end of each digit.
3. Pollex
4. Miniature long bone
5. Head; base
6. 5
7. The wrist
8. Lateral
9. Head of the metacarpals
10. 8
11. Trapezium, trapezoid, capitate, hamate
12. Triquetrum
13. Capitate; os magnum
14. Lunate
15. Navicular; lateral
16. Because unciform means hook-shaped and the hamate has a hooklike process on it
17. Trapezium; greater multangular
18. It is located on the proximal row of the carpal bones on the anteromedial side of the wrist.
19. Anterior
20. Radius and ulna
21. Radius
22. 1st–5th metacarpals
23. Radius, ulna, and humerus
24. Proximal; distal

25. At the distal end of the ulna, on the medial side of the ulnar head
26. Short
27. Radius
28. Ulna
29. Diaphyses
30. Extended
31. Radial notch
32. The trochlear (semilunar) notch is the large concave depression on the anterior side of the ulna between the coronoid process and the olecranon process.
33. Proximal
34. Olecranon and coronoid processes
35. Coronoid
36. Radius; ulna
37. Condyle
38. Coronoid fossa, olecranon fossa, and radial fossa
39. Deltoid tuberosity
40. Anatomical; surgical
41. Phalanges; carpals
42. Capitulum; capitellum
43. Trochlea; trochlear (semilunar) notch
44. Lateral; anteromedial
45. Intertubercular (bicipital) groove
46. Medial epicondyle
47. The trochlear sulcus is the constricted central area of the trochlea on the distal humerus.
48. Medial epicondyle; when it is bumped, a painful or tingling sensation is felt in the arm due to the presence of the ulnar nerve on its posterior side.
49. Synovial; diarthrodial
50. Surgical neck
51. Proximal interphalangeal joint
52. 1st metacarpophalangeal joints and 1st carpometacarpal joints of the right and left hands
53. Glenohumeral
54. Diarthrodial; ball and socket
55. Proximal and distal radioulnar joints
56. Capitulum (capitellum)
57. Radiocarpal joint
58. Gliding
59. Hinge
60. Humeroradial joint is formed between the capitulum of the humerus and the head of the radius; the humero-ulnar joint is formed between the trochlea of the humerus and trochlear notch of the ulna.
61. Interphalangeal joint of the 1st digit of the left hand
62. 3rd metacarpophalangeal joint of the left hand
63. P
64. G
65. H
66. S
67. C
68. S
69. B
70. G
71. H
72. C
73. The splint and bandage should only be removed with the physician's permission. An initial set of radiographs may be taken with the splint in place to determine the presence and severity of a fracture. The physician may then request that the splint be removed and the radiographs repeated.

74. When more than one projection is taken on a film, lead masking can shield the unexposed side from scatter radiation; it can also aid in accurate part centering on one half of the cassette.

75. The shoulder should lie on the same plane as the wrist so that the elbow joint is in a true lateral position. If the shoulder is higher than the elbow, the humeral epicondyles will not be superimposed.

76. AP and lateral

77. PA, oblique, and lateral

78. Since there are many small bones in the wrist, it is difficult to see minute fractures. The detail on the radiograph will be greater if a slow speed film/screen combination is used. Since the single humerus is a much larger bone than the carpals, it is easier to see pathology on it without the aid of detail cassettes.

79. Proximal interphalangeal (PIP) joint

80. 50 kVp

81. Distal ⅓ of the metacarpal

82. The metacarpals and phalanges of the 2nd through 5th digits should exhibit symmetrical curvatures on the medial and lateral sides and the thumb should lie in an oblique position.

83. Proximal and distal interphalangeal joints and metacarpophalangeal joint

84. 45°

85. Rotate the hand internally to place the 2nd digit in direct contact with the cassette.

86. Lateral

87. Soft tissue should be evident; the cortex and trabeculae should be visualized and sharp.

88. The hand is in an AP position when supinated; if the hand is pronated, the radius crosses the ulna.

89. 3rd metacarpophalangeal joint

90. The fingers were not positioned parallel to the film plane. Perhaps a radiolucent step sponge was not used to assist in patient positioning.

91. Lateral

92. Arching the hand and resting the fingertips on the cassette will minimize the OID and distortion of the carpals.

93. PA oblique and PA wrist in ulnar flexion

94. 45°

95. The elbow is flexed 90° and placed flat on the surface of the cassette.

96. 25–30°; 3rd metacarpal

97. One-third

98. To adequately demonstrate the entire elbow joint and adjacent structures, two projections must be taken. Placing the forearm on the cassette will demonstrate the proximal radius and ulna and placing the humerus on the cassette will demonstrate the distal humerus, epicondyles, and condyles with capitulum and trochlea.

99. 60–65 kVp

100. 45°

101. The proximal radioulnar joint should be open and demonstrated. The capitulum of the humerus should also be well demonstrated.

102. The radial head is mostly superimposed over the coronoid process of the ulna. An axial lateral projection will present an elongated view of the radial head free of superimposition.

103. The epicondyles of the humerus are superimposed; the trochlea and capitulum are superimposed and appear cylindrical. The trochlea is demonstrated in the trochlear notch of the ulna.

104. Lateral

105. AP and lateral

106. Neutral AP and transthoracic lateral

107. A breathing technique (long exposure time) will result in blurring of the ribs and lung markings that overlie the humerus.

108. Oblique projection of the hand

109. Tangential carpal canal projection of the wrist

110. AP projection of the forearm

111. Medial (internal) oblique projection of the elbow

112. Lateral projection of the humerus

113.

Projection	CR Angle/ Angle of Part	Centering Point	Film Size	Structures Seen
Lateral hand	CR = no angle Part = 90°	MCP joints	8×10 in. lw	2nd–5th metacarpals superimposed; carpals superimposed; phalanges superimposed on extension but separated on fan lateral; thumb in PA projection
Transthoracic lateral humerus	CR = horizontal beam part = 90° from neutral AP	Surgical neck of humerus	10×12 in. lw or 11×14 in. lw	Head, surgical neck, and proximal ⅔ of humerus seen between spine and sternum; glenoid cavity of scapula also demonstrated
PA wrist	CR = no angle part = no rotation	Midcarpal region	8×10 in. cw or 10×12 in. cw	Carpal bones, particularly the scaphoid, lunate, capitate, trapezium, and hamate. 2 in. of distal forearm and proximal metacarpals also included
Lateral forearm	CR = no angle part = 90°	Midway between humeral epicondyles and radiocarpal joint	10×12 in. lw or 11×14 in. lw	Shafts of radius and ulna separated; radial tuberosity directed anteriorly; olecranon process of ulna in profile, radial head partly superimposed over coronoid process of ulna. 2 in. of distal humerus, carpals, and proximal metacarpals included

DISCUSSION OF ATYPICAL CASE STUDIES ◄

1. The patient who sewed through her thumb with an industrial sewing machine should be left on the stretcher due to her physical condition. The three radiographs usually ordered are the AP, PA oblique, and lateral. In this case, it may be better to radiograph the thumb using a PA projection. The hand should be propped up and steadied so the thumb would not be resting on the needle.

2. Since the left hand and wrist are normally radiographed for a bone age study, this case involving the child with an abnormal left hand presents a bit of a dilemma. If bone age films have been done previously, the same parts should be visualized so a comparison can be made. If there are no previous films a radiologist should be consulted if available. Most likely you would be directed to radiograph the right hand and wrist as this would give the radiologist the most information.

3. An AP projection radiograph would work the best for the patient whose wrist is casted in a flexed position. The technique increase would be minimal for the fiberglass cast and all the positions/projections should be performed using regular or fast speed screens.

4. The AP would be requested because the radius crosses over the ulna when the hand is pronated and in this case may obscure the fracture site. If the patient's plaster cast is wet, the mAs should be doubled. These positions/projections should also be performed using regular or fast speed screens.

5. For the patient who cannot extend his elbow, two AP radiographs should be performed. One radiograph with the radius/ulna parallel to the cassette, and one radiograph with the humerus parallel to the cassette. The obliques could be attempted with the elbow flexed, although if it is not discouraged by the clinical site, an axial lateral elbow could be substituted for the external oblique.

6. The radiograph that would visualize the radial head free of superimposition on the boy who fell roller skating is the external oblique. The axial lateral elbow would also visualize this part.

7. The large foam wedge positioned between the patient's arm and thorax should not be removed for the two humerus radiographs. For the two views 90° apart, one radiograph could be obtained with the patient facing an upright Bucky. The projection would be PA although since the humeral epicondyles would be approximately perpendicular to the film, this would achieve a lateral radiograph of the humerus. The patient then could be turned laterally and a radiograph taken with the epicondyles approximately parallel for the second radiograph.

SHOULDER GIRDLE 6

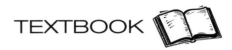

TEXTBOOK

Objectives

Following the completion of this chapter, the student will be able to:

1. Given diagrams, radiographs, or dry bones, name and describe the bones of the shoulder girdle, to include the scapula, clavicle, and proximal humerus.
2. Describe the relationship of the structures on the shoulder girdle (ie, the coracoid process is anterior and medial to the glenoid fossa).
3. Classify the articulations of the shoulder girdle and identify their type of movement.
4. Describe patient preparation and care relative to radiographic examination of the shoulder girdle.
5. Describe alternative projections for demonstrating the glenohumeral relationship.
6. List and describe the basic projections of the shoulder girdle, to include preferred type and size of image receptor, central ray location, and structures best visualized.
7. Discuss the breathing instructions for radiographic examinations of the shoulder girdle.
8. Practice positioning the basic projections of the shoulder girdle on another student or phantom.
9. Describe procedural modifications for patients suspected of having a humeral fracture.
10. State the criteria used to determine positioning accuracy on radiographs of the shoulder girdle.
11. Evaluate radiographs of the shoulder girdle in terms of positioning, centering, image quality, radiographic anatomy, and pathology.
12. Define terminology associated with the shoulder girdle, to include anatomy, procedures, and pathology.
13. Identify the reason(s) for radiographing the AC joints in the erect position and taking radiographs with and without weights.
14. Describe equipment considerations and exposure factors relative to radiography of the shoulder girdle.

Chapter Outline

   I. ANATOMY OF THE SHOULDER GIRDLE
      A. Clavicle
      B. Scapula
  II. ARTHROLOGY OF THE SHOULDER GIRDLE
      A. Acromioclavicular Joint
      B. Sternoclavicular Joint
      C. Glenohumeral Joint

III. PROCEDURAL CONSIDERATIONS
    A. Patient Preparations
    B. Positioning Considerations
    C. Alternate Projections
    D. Breathing Instructions
    E. Exposure Factors
    F. Equipment Considerations

IV. RADIOGRAPHIC POSITIONING OF THE SHOULDER GIRDLE
    A. Shoulder: AP in External Rotation, AP in Internal Rotation, Inferosuperior Axial, PA Oblique "Y"
        1. technical considerations
        2. shielding
        3. patient positioning
        4. part positioning
        5. central ray
        6. breathing instructions
        7. image evaluation
        8. critical anatomy
    B. Clavicle: AP, AP Axial
        1. technical considerations
        2. shielding
        3. patient positioning
        4. part positioning
        5. central ray
        6. breathing instructions
        7. image evaluation
        8. critical anatomy
    C. Scapula: AP, Lateral
        1. technical considerations
        2. shielding
        3. patient positioning
        4. part positioning
        5. central ray
        6. breathing instructions
        7. image evaluation
        8. critical anatomy
    D. Acromioclavicular Joints: AP With and Without Weights
        1. technical considerations
        2. shielding
        3. patient positioning
        4. part positioning
        5. central ray
        6. breathing instructions
        7. image evaluation
        8. critical anatomy

V. SUMMARY
VI. CRITICAL THINKING & APPLICATION QUESTIONS
VII. FILM CRITIQUE

SAMPLE 50-MINUTE LESSON ◄

PREPARATION STEP

ESTIMATED TIME—10 MINUTES

A. Assemble teaching aids
1. Overhead projector
2. Overhead transparencies
   a. included in *Instructor's Resource Manual*
   b. trace drawings from *Applications Manual* on clear radiographic film
3. Skeleton
4. Radiographs
B. Introduce topics of articulations and procedural considerations for the shoulder girdle. Lecture will include Chapter Objectives 3, 4, and 5.
C. Opening discussion
1. The basic anatomy was discussed during the last class. We will be continuing with the objectives beginning with the joints of the shoulder girdle. We will then continue with procedural considerations for positioning of this area.

PRESENTATION STEP

ESTIMATED TIME—40 MINUTES

TEACHING OUTLINE	TEACHING AIDS & METHODS
I. Arthrology of the Shoulder Girdle	*Transparency of joints*
A. Sternoclavicular Joint	
1. synovial joint	
2. diarthrodial gliding	
3. where clavicle articulates with axial skeleton	
B. Acromioclavicular Joint	
1. synovial joint	
2. diarthrodial gliding	
3. only articulation between the bones of the shoulder girdle	
C. Glenohumeral Joint (Shoulder)	
1. synovial joint	
2. diarthrodial ball and socket: wide range of movement but relatively unstable because glenoid fossa is so shallow	
II. Procedural Considerations	
A. Patient Preparation	
1. first check to be sure correct patient	
2. remove all clothing and jewelry from the waist up	
3. if patient's arm is in a sling it should not be removed without physician approval	*Demonstrate having arm in a sling*
4. relevant patient history is essential as projections depend on reason for examination	
B. Positioning Considerations	*Radiographic examples*
1. shoulder	
a. nontraumatic shoulder examinations usually include two AP projections	
(1) external/internal rotation	
(2) patient can be positioned supine, sitting, or standing	
b. possible fracture	

(1) do not move arm as may cause additional damage to muscles, vessels, or nerves

(2) take two projections 90° apart
    (a) neutral AP and transthoracic

(3) perform with patient in upright position when possible as this is more comfortable for the patient

  2. clavicle
    a. lateral projection would not be helpful in identifying pathology
    b. two projections would be AP or PA and axial

  3. scapula
    a. AP and lateral with patient recumbent or upright
    b. abduct arm for AP projection to pull scapula out from under rib cage

  4. acromioclavicular joints
    a. done to evaluate soft tissue damage evidenced by increased joint separation when weights used to apply gentle pressure traction
    b. always bilateral study with and without weights
    c. patient always in upright position
    d. 72 in. SID is used to minimize magnification so both will fit

III. Alternate Projections
  A. Lateral Scapular Plane Position—"Y" View
    1. 45–60° LAO or RAO upright
    2. beneficial to assess dislocation
  B. Inferosuperior Axial Projection
    1. demonstrates relationship of glenoid fossa and radial head
  C. Transthoracic
    1. demonstrates displacement of fracture fragments and glenohumeral relationship

IV. Breathing Instructions
  A. Shoulder and AP Clavicle—Stop Breathing
  B. Axial Clavicle—Inspiration to Elevate Clavicle
  C. AP Scapula—Breathing Technique to Blur Out Rib Detail
  D. AC Joints—Expiration as Relaxes Shoulders

V. Exposure Factors
  A. 60–75 kVp/Grid
  B. Lower kVp for Patients With Decreased Bone Mass (ie, Osteoporosis)
  C. Higher kVp for Muscular Patients

VI. Equipment Consideration
  A. Shoulders Most Often Done With a Grid
  B. Mobile Radiography Often Does Not Use a Grid to Avoid Possible Grid Lines and Reduce Patient Exposure

Radiographic examples

● **APPLICATION STEP**   ESTIMATED TIME—2 HOURS

Study Assignment

A. Continue reading Chapter 6 in the text.
B. Find all the anatomy discussed on the skeleton.
C. Find all the anatomy discussed on the radiographs of the shoulder girdle.
D. Continue Chapter 6 in the *Applications Manual.*
E. Compare the positioning drawings in the *Applications Manual* to a corresponding radiograph.
F. Critique radiographs for image quality and proper positioning. Be sure you can locate the anatomic parts listed on the drawing worksheets on each of the radiographs.

TESTING STEP

Questions on this material will be included in exam given at end of this chapter.

EXAM QUESTIONS ◄

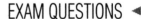

Multiple Choice

1. You are looking at two unmarked shoulder films. How can you tell in which radiograph the humerus is externally rotated and in which radiograph the humerus is internally rotated?
   A. the external rotation shows the humeral head as smooth and round
   B. the internal rotation shows the lesser tuberosity on the lateral side of the humeral head
   C. the external rotation shows the greater tuberosity in profile
   D. the internal rotation shows the bicipital groove in profile

2. When radiographing the acromion and coronoid processes of the lateral scapula, where should the patient's affected arm be positioned if possible?
   A. extended above the head with the forearm resting on the head or opposite shoulder
   B. hanging on the side in a neutral position
   C. resting in the patient's lap
   D. none of the above

3. What two shoulder radiographs would you take if the patient has a possible surgical neck fracture?
   A. internal and external rotation of the shoulder
   B. external rotation and transthoracic
   C. "Y" view and inferosuperior axial
   D. internal rotation and "Y" view

4. How should the patient be positioned when performing the radiograph for possible AC joint separation?
   A. prone
   B. supine
   C. upright
   D. lateral

5. Which margin of the scapula is proximal to the axilla?
   A. superior
   B. inferior
   C. medial
   D. lateral

6. When viewed from a lateral perspective, what parts of the scapula form the "Y"?
   A. body, acromion process, coracoid process
   B. glenoid fossa, coronoid process, spine
   C. supraspinous fossa, infraspinous fossa, spine
   D. AC joint, SC joint, glenohumeral joint

7. On the PA oblique "Y" radiograph of the shoulder, if the humerus were dislocated anteriorly where would it be visualized?
   A. under the acromion process
   B. under the coracoid process
   C. under the coronoid process
   D. in the glenoid cavity

8. Which anatomic part is radiographed to evaluate soft-tissue damage evidenced by increased joint separation when weights are applied to the patient's wrists?
   A. AP neutral shoulder
   B. AP internal shoulder
   C. PA clavicle
   D. AC joints

9. Why is it important for an exposure of AC joints to be done on expiration?
   A. the lung markings will be blurred out
   B. when exhaling the shoulders and arms relax, allowing for better assessment of any joint separation
   C. expiration elevates the clavicles for better separation
   D. the patient will be more at ease, making for a better radiograph

10. What three anatomical parts are seen on an appropriately positioned and well-penetrated inferosuperior shoulder radiograph?
    A. coracoid process, clavicle, SC articulation
    B. coronoid process, humeral head, bicipital groove
    C. acromion process, humeral head, glenoid cavity
    D. acromion process, sternal extremity of the clavicle, glenoid cavity

11. Which radiograph visualizes the relationship between the glenoid cavity and the humeral head?
    1. transthoracic
    2. inferosuperior axial projection
    3. PA oblique "Y"
       A. 1 only
       B. 2 and 3 only
       C. 1 and 3 only
       D. 1, 2, and 3

ANSWER KEY

1. C	4. C	7. B	10. C
2. A	5. D	8. D	11. D
3. D	6. A	9. B	

APPLICATIONS MANUAL

DRAWINGS ◄

The same directions apply to the drawings in this unit. Each bone should be colored a different color and the appropriate parts should be labeled.

ANSWER KEY FOR STUDY QUESTIONS ◄

1. Scapula and clavicle
2. The shoulder girdle attaches the bones of the upper limb to the axial skeleton.
3. Scapula
4. The sternoclavicular joint
5. Collarbone; shoulder blade
6. Long; flat
7. Sternal end (extremity); acromial end (extremity)
8. Shaft
9. Acromial end
10. The medial ⅔ of the clavicle is convex forward, while the lateral ⅓ is concave forward.
11. Conoid tubercle
12. The clavicle limits the movement of the shoulder girdle and aids in preventing a dislocation of the shoulder.
13. Males
14. Triangular-shaped
15. 2nd; 7th
16. Lateral, medial (vertebral), and superior borders
17. Lateral
18. It is the central area or body of the scapula.
19. Ventral; costal
20. Ventral (anterior)
21. Dorsal (posterior)
22. Acromion
23. Coracoid process
24. The scapular notch is located at the base of the coracoid process on its medial side on the superior border of the scapula.
25. Interior
26. Lateral
27. Glenoid cavity
28. The acromion of the scapula and the clavicle form the acromioclavicular joint.
29. Superior
30. Supraspinous and infraspinous fossae

31. Glenoid cavity
32. Coracoid process
33. Subscapular fossa
34. Coracoid process of the scapula and the conoid tubercle of the clavicle
35. When viewed from the side, the acromion and corocoid process form the upper extension and the body forms the lower vertical portion of the Y.
36. Synovial; diarthrodial
37. Three
38. Glenohumeral joint
39. Diarthrodial; ball and socket
40. Gliding
41. Acromioclavicular
42. Separation injury
43. Head of the humerus and the glenoid cavity of the scapula
44. Gliding
45. Shoulder joint (glenohumeral)
46. Removal of all clothing and jewelry from the waist up
47. Either PA and PA axial or AP and AP axial projections
48. AP erect projections—weight-bearing and nonweight-bearing
49. Fracture fragments could cause additional damage to muscles, vessels, or nerves.
50. Abduction of the arm helps pull the scapula out from under the rib cage.
51. Neutral AP and transthoracic lateral projections
52. 5–10 lb
53. 60 kVp is recommended for very small patients, especially osteoporotic patients; 75 kVp might be necessary to penetrate extremely muscular patients.
54. To minimize magnification and increase the probability of including both joints on the same film
55. PA oblique "Y" and transthoracic lateral projections
56. The exam is performed as a bilateral study so that the injured joint can be compared to the uninjured joint to evaluate the extent of a separation injury.
57. Suspended expiration; because the shoulders and arms are more likely to relax downward when a person exhales
58. Separate nonweight-bearing and weight-bearing exposures of each joint must be taken individually on small cassettes.
59. The shoulder and clavicle series must be completed first in order to rule out fractures. Once they have been cleared by the physician, the AC joints can be radiographed.
60. The hand is in supination.
61. Coracoid process
62. AP projection of the shoulder in external rotation
63. AP projection of the shoulder in internal rotation
64. Glenohumeral joint
65. The CR is directed horizontally and medially through the axilla to the AC joint; the amount of medial angulation generally ranges from 15 to 30°.
66. 45–60°
67. The head of the humerus is dislocated from the glenoid cavity. In an anterior dislocation, the humeral head will be situated under the coracoid process of the scapula on the PA oblique "Y" projection.
68. The CR should be angled approximately 15–30° caudally. The degree of the angle depends upon the patient's size. A smaller patient will require a greater degree of angulation than a larger patient.
69. Inspiration because it elevates the clavicle
70. False; the scapula can be radiographed in the upright or recumbent position.
71. True
72. False; a sling should never be removed without prior approval from a physician. The shoulder can be radiographed with the sling in place.

73. False; in the lateral position, the ribs and lungs do not overlie the scapula.
74. False; even with the arm abducted 90° from the body, the medial half of the scapula will lie under the bony thorax.
75.

Projection	CR Angle/Angle of Part	Centering Point	Film Size	Structures Seen
AP shoulder in internal rotation74	CR = perpendicular part = internal rotation	Coracoid process of scapula	10×12 in. lw or cw	Lesser tubercle of humerus in profile against the glenoid cavity of scapula; greater tubercle superimposed over humeral head
PA oblique "Y" shoulder	CR = perpendicular part = midcoronal plane rotated 45–60° to film plane	Through midpoint of vertebral border of scapula to the glenohumeral joint	10×12 in. lw	Relationship of humeral head with the glenoid cavity of the scapula (demonstrates anterior and posterior dislocations)
AP axial clavicle	CR = 25–30° cephalad	Midpoint of clavicle	10×12 in. cw	Majority projected above the ribs and chest with the medial end superimposed over the 1st and 2nd ribs
Lateral scapula	CR = perpendicular part = approx. 45–60° rotation until body of scapula is perpendicular to film plane	Vertebral border of scapula between the acromion and inferior angle	10×12 in. lw	Body of scapula free of superimposition on rib cage; acromion and coracoid process; costal and dorsal surfaces
AP AC joints with weights	CR = perpendicular and horizontally at 72 in. SID part = 0°	Bilateral exam: midway between the AC joints on midsagittal plane	14×17 in. cw or 7×17 in. cw	Joint space of both AC joints should be demonstrated; joints will be asymetrical if separation is present.

DISCUSSION OF ATYPICAL CASE STUDIES ◄

1. The two radiographs 90° apart of the proximal humerus could be accomplished in two basic ways. The most common way would be to do an AP neutral shoulder radiograph and a transthoracic radiograph. An alternate approach would be to do the AP neutral shoulder radiograph with the patient obliqued approximately 45° toward the side of interest and a PA oblique "Y" view with the patient obliqued approximately 45° toward the side of interest.

2. The AP scapula on the heavily sedated woman would be performed in the usual manner with her arm abducted at a 90° angle to her body. The lateral would have to be done using an AP projection rather than the usual PA. The patient should be rolled up away from the side of interest and her arm should be manipulated as well as possible to move the humerus away from the scapular body.

3. Since the patient in this case study does not want to turn his back toward you, the clavicle radiographs will have to be performed using an AP projection. A cephalic angle should be used if the projection is an AP.

4. The best way to radiograph the football player's AC joints would be to place two 8 × 10 films in a film holder so you would have 20 in. in which to fit the AC joints rather than 17 in. Doing them simultaneously if possible is still best. If this approach is not feasible, then each joint could be done separately. Four exposures would be necessary for this approach.

LOWER LIMB (EXTREMITY) 7

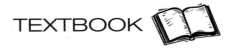

TEXTBOOK

Objectives

Following the completion of this chapter, the student will be able to:

1. Given diagrams, radiographs, or dry bones, name and describe the bones of the lower limb, to include the foot, ankle, lower leg, knee, and femur.
2. Identify any surface markings found on the bones of the lower limb.
3. List any additional names for the bones, structures, or surfaces of the lower limb, especially the foot.
4. Locate the transverse and longitudinal arches in each foot and discuss their function.
5. Classify the articulations in the lower limb and identify their type of movement.
6. List and describe the basic projections of the lower limb, to include preferred size of image receptor, central ray location, and structures best visualized.
7. Describe the positioning steps for taking supplemental projections of the lower limb due to trauma, pain, etc.
8. Practice positioning the basic projections of the lower limb on another student or phantom.
9. State the criteria used to determine positioning accuracy on radiographs of the lower limb.
10. Evaluate radiographs of the lower limb in terms of positioning, centering, image quality, radiographic anatomy, and pathology.
11. Describe equipment considerations and exposure factors relative to radiography of the lower limb.
12. Define terminology associated with the lower limb, to include anatomy, procedures, and pathology.

Chapter Outline

I. ANATOMY OF THE LOWER LIMB
   A. Foot and Ankle
      1. phalanges
      2. metatarsals
      3. tarsals
   B. Arches of the Foot
   C. Lower Leg
      1. tibia

    D. Upper Leg
      1. femur
    E. Kneecap
      1. patella

II. ARTHROLOGY OF THE LOWER LIMB
    A. Interphalangeal Joints
    B. Metatarsophalangeal Joints
    C. Intermetatarsal Joints
    D. Tarsometatarsal Joints
    E. Intertarsal Joints
    F. Ankle Joint
      1. tibiotalar
      2. fibulotalar
    G. Distal Tibiofibular Joint
    H. Proximal Tibiofibular Joint
    I. Knee
      1. tibiofemoral
      2. femoropatellar
    J. Hip

III. PROCEDURAL CONSIDERATIONS
    A. Patient Preparations
    B. Positioning Considerations
    C. Alternate Projections
    D. Pediatric Radiography
    E. Exposure Factors
    F. Equipment Considerations

IV. RADIOGRAPHIC POSITIONING OF THE LOWER LIMB
    A. Toes: AP, Medial Oblique, Lateral
      1. technical considerations
      2. shielding
      3. patient positioning
      4. part positioning
      5. central ray
      6. image evaluation
      7. critical anatomy
    B. Sesamoids: Tangential Metatarsophalangeal
      1. technical considerations
      2. shielding
      3. patient positioning
      4. part positioning
      5. central ray
      6. image evaluation
      7. critical anatomy
    C. Foot: AP, Medial Oblique, Lateral
      1. technical considerations
      2. shielding
      3. patient positioning

      4. part positioning

      5. central ray

      6. image evaluation

      7. critical anatomy

  D. Calcaneus (Os Calcis): Axial Plantodorsal, Lateral

      1. technical considerations

      2. shielding

      3. patient positioning

      4. part positioning

      5. central ray

      6. image evaluation

      7. critical anatomy

  E. Ankle: AP, Medial Oblique, Lateral

      1. technical considerations

      2. shielding

      3. patient positioning

      4. part positioning

      5. central ray

      6. image evaluation

      7. critical anatomy

  F. Lower Leg: AP, Lateral

      1. technical considerations

      2. shielding

      3. patient positioning

      4. part positioning

      5. central ray

      6. image evaluation

      7. critical anatomy

  G. Knee: AP, Medial Oblique, Lateral Oblique, Lateral, PA Axial Intercondylar Fossa (Camp–Coventry Method), PA Axial Intercondylar Fossa (Homblad Method)

      1. technical considerations

      2. shielding

      3. patient positioning

      4. part positioning

      5. central ray

      6. image evaluation

      7. critical anatomy

  H. Patella: PA, Lateral, Tangential

      1. technical considerations

      2. shielding

      3. patient positioning

      4. part positioning

      5. central ray

      6. image evaluation

      7. critical anatomy

I. Femur: AP, Lateral
   1. technical considerations
   2. shielding
   3. patient positioning
   4. part positioning
   5. central ray
   6. image evaluation
   7. critical anatomy
V. SUMMARY
VI. CRITICAL THINKING & APPLICATION QUESTIONS
VII. FILM CRITIQUE

► SAMPLE 50-MINUTE LESSON

PREPARATION STEP

ESTIMATED TIME—10 MINUTES

A. Assemble teaching aids
   1. Overhead projector
   2. Overhead transparencies
      a. included in *Instructor's Resource Manual*
      b. trace drawings from *Applications Manual* on clear radiographic film
   3. Skeleton
   4. Radiographs
B. Introduce topics of positioning of the lower limb. Lecture will include Chapter Objectives 6 and 7.
C. Opening discussion
   1. Anatomy and procedural considerations have been presented. This lecture will continue with the positioning for basic and supplemental projections of the lower limb.
   2. This lecture will cover the positioning of toes, feet, and calcaneous.
   3. Be sure you can visualize the anatomy that is seen on each projection or position discussed.
   4. All children and adults of reproductive age should be shielded for all radiographic exams of the lower extremity. The patient should be asked not to move during the exposure as breathing instructions are not important. The SID for the majority of lower extremity radiographs is 40 in.; any exceptions will be noted when the position/projection is covered.

PRESENTATION STEP

ESTIMATED TIME—40 MINUTES

TEACHING OUTLINE	TEACHING AIDS & METHODS
I. Positioning of the Lower Limb	*Transparency of lower limb*
A. AP Toes	
1. technical considerations	
2. 8 × 10 in.	*Radiograph of toes*
a. detail/extremity cassette	
b. table top	
3. positioning	
a. plantar surface of foot on cassette	
4. central ray	
a. perpendicular to second metatarsophalangeal joint or to individual toe MP joint	

     5. structures visualized
       a. bony and soft tissue structures of toe and distal
        metatarsal

B. Medial Oblique Toes
  1. technical considerations   *Radiograph of toes*
    a. 8 × 10 in.
    b. detail/extremity cassette
    c. table top
  2. positioning
    a. internally rotate leg and foot until plantar sur-
       face forms 30° angle to film
  3. central ray
    a. perpendicular to second metatarsophalangeal
       joint or to individual toe MP joint
  4. structures visualized
    a. bony and soft tissue structures of toe and distal
       metatarsal

C. Lateral Toes
  1. technical considerations   *Radiograph of toes*
    a. 8 × 10 in.
    b. detail/extremity cassette
    c. table top
  2. positioning
    a. rotate leg medially or laterally depending on
       which toe
    b. separate toes to prevent superimposition
  3. central ray
    a. perpendicular to cassette through IP or PIP
  4. structures visualized
    a. bony and soft tissue structures of toe and distal
       metatarsal

D. Tangential Metatarsophalangeal Sesamoids
  1. technical considerations   *Radiograph*
    a. 8 × 10 in.
    b. detail/extremity cassette
    c. table top
  2. positioning   *Demonstrate position*
    a. kneeling or prone position
    b. dorsiflex foot and MP joints until plantar sur-
       face of toes rests firmly on cassette
  3. central ray
    a. perpendicular to cassette through 1st MP joint
  4. structures visualized
    a. sesamoid bones and joint spaces between ses-
       amoids and distal metatarsals

E. AP Foot
  1. technical considerations   *Foot radiographs*
    a. 10 × 12 in.
    b. detail/extremity cassette
    c. table top
  2. positioning
    a. plantar surface of foot on cassette

3. central ray
    a. 5–15° posterior angle depending on longitudinal arch of foot
    b. center through base of 3rd metatarsal
4. structures visualized
    a. bony and soft tissue structures from toes to tarsals
    b. phalanges, metatarsals, tarsals anterior to talus

F. Medial Oblique Foot
  1. technical considerations   *Foot radiographs*
    a. 10 × 12 in.
    b. detail/extremity cassette
    c. table top
  2. positioning
    a. internally rotate leg and foot until plantar surface forms 30° angle with plane of cassette
  3. central ray
    a. perpendicular to cassette through base of 3rd metatarsal
  4. structures visualized
    a. bony and soft tissue structures from toes to tarsals
    b. phalanges, metatarsals, cuneiforms, and navicular
    c. 3rd–5th MP joints
    d. base of 5th metatarsal

G. Lateral Foot
  1. technical considerations   *Foot radiographs*
    a. 10 × 12 in.
    b. detail/extremity cassette
    c. table top
  2. positioning
    a. laterally rotate foot until plantar surface is perpendicular to cassette
    b. elevate knee until patella is perpendicular to cassette
  3. central ray
    a. perpendicular to cassette through tarsometatarsal joints
  4. structures visualized
    a. bony and soft tissue structures from toes to tarsals
    b. superimposed phalanges and metatarsals, calcaneus, talus, navicular, ankle joint, and 1 in. of distal tibia and fibula

H. Axial Plantodorsal Calcaneus (Os Calcis)
  1. technical considerations   *Calcaneus radiographs*
    a. 8 × 10 in. or 10 × 12 in.
    b. detail/extremity cassette
    c. table top
  2. positioning
    a. dorsiflex foot so plantar surface is perpendicular to cassette at 90° angle
    b. patient may need to gently pull back foot with tape or gauze

3. central ray
   a. 40° cephalic angle centered to midplantar surface at the level of the base of 5th metatarsal
4. structures visualized
   a. bony and soft tissue structures
   b. calcaneus, sustentaculum tali, tuberosity, trochlear process, and subtalor joint

I. Lateral Calcaneus (Os Calcis)
1. technical considerations
   a. 8 × 10 in. or 10 × 12 in.
   b. detail/extremity cassette
   c. table top
2. patient positioning
   a. laterally rotate foot until plantar surface is perpendicular to cassette
   b. elevate knee until patella is perpendicular to cassette
3. central ray
   a. perpendicular to cassette through a point 1–1½ in. distal to the medial malleolus
4. structures visualized
   a. bony and soft tissue structures
   b. calcaneus, talus, navicular, tuberosity in profile and sinus tarsi

APPLICATION STEP

ESTIMATED TIME—2 HOURS

Study Assignment

A. Continue reading Chapter 7 in the text.
B. Continue Chapter 7 in the *Applications Manual.*
C. Compare the positioning drawings in the *Applications Manual* to a corresponding radiograph.
D. Critique radiographs for image quality and proper positioning. Be sure you can locate the anatomic parts listed on the drawing worksheets on each of the radiographs.

TESTING STEP

Questions on this material will be included in exam given at end of this chapter.

EXAM QUESTIONS ◄

Multiple Choice

1. Which position/projection BEST demonstrates the cuboid, 3rd cuneiform, and the base of the 3rd metatarsal?
   A. weight-bearing lateral foot
   B. AP foot
   C. medial oblique foot
   D. lateral oblique foot

2. Where should the CR be centered on an AP ankle projection, if the hospital protocol states that as much of the tibia/fibula as possible should be included on the radiograph?
   A. centered between the knee and ankle
   B. on the ankle joint
   C. 4 in. proximal to the ankle joint
   D. on whichever part of the leg is in the middle of the cassette

3. What is the purpose of angling the CR 5° cephalad on a lateral projection of the knee?
   A. it prevents superimposition of the joint space by the medial condyle
   B. it prevents superimposition of the joint space by the lateral condyle
   C. it helps visualize the patella in profile
   D. it opens up the joint space between the femur and patella

4. What is the purpose of using a 48 in. SID when radiographing a lower leg diagonally on a 14 × 17 in. cassette?
   A. so the divergent rays will open up the ankle joint
   B. so the divergent rays will open up the knee joint
   C. so the ankle and knee will both be included in the collimated area visualized on the radiograph
   D. so the ankle and knee will physically fit on the cassette

5. The radiograph was taken with the knee rotated 45° medially. The patient is supine. What main structure is visualized?
   A. tibial tuberosity in profile
   B. the femoropatellar joint space opened up
   C. the fibula superimposed over the proximal tibia
   D. the head and neck of the fibula and proximal tib-fib articulation

6. The radiograph was taken with the knee rotated 45° laterally. The patient is prone. What main structure is visualized?
   A. tibial tuberosity in profile
   B. the femoropatellar joint space opened up
   C. the fibula superimposed over the proximal tibia
   D. the head and neck of the fibula and proximal tib-fib articulation

7. Which position/projection best visualizes the tibial tuberosity in profile?
   A. lateral knee
   B. AP knee
   C. medial oblique knee
   D. lateral oblique knee

8. What condition occurs when the ligaments and tendons of the longitudinal arches are excessively strained and weakened?
   A. bunions
   B. pes planus
   C. gout
   D. tendonitis

9. On which position is it imperative to include the base of the 5th metatarsal?
   A. AP ankle
   B. medial oblique ankle
   C. lateral ankle
   D. plantodorsal calcaneus

10. If the proximal fibula is fractured as the result of a twisting type of injury, it is highly probable that there will be another fracture on the
    A. patella
    B. distal fibula
    C. proximal tibia
    D. distal tibia

11. On an AP ankle radiograph which malleolus visualizes as more inferior?
    A. medial
    B. lateral
    C. posterior
    D. anterior

12. Where is the femur located on a patient who has excess adipose tissue on the thighs?
    A. anteriorly and medially
    B. anteriorly and laterally
    C. posteriorly and medially
    D. posteriorly and laterally

13. What procedure is used to assist in identification of possible partial or complete tears of the ligaments of the ankle?
    A. an AP ankle and lateral ankle radiograph is obtained
    B. a medial oblique and lateral oblique ankle radiograph is obtained
    C. the physician inverts or everts the foot while a radiograph is obtained
    D. the patient is asked to stand and bear all his/her weight on the affected ankle

14. What type of radiograph is often taken to evaluate degenerative arthritis in the knee?
    A. weight-bearing AP bilateral projections of the knees
    B. recumbent bilateral lateral knees
    C. medial and lateral oblique knees
    D. recumbent bilateral intercondylar fossa radiographs

15. What amount of angulation of the CR should be used when attaining weight-bearing AP bilateral projections of the knees?
    A. the central ray is horizontal and no angulation is used
    B. the central ray is angled 5° cephalad
    C. the central ray is angled 15° cephalad
    D. the central ray is angled 25° cephalad

Answer Key

1. C	4. C	7. A	10. D	13. C
2. B	5. D	8. B	11. B	14. A
3. A	6. D	9. C	12. B	15. A

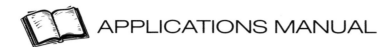 APPLICATIONS MANUAL

▶ DRAWINGS

The same directions apply to the drawings in this unit. Each bone should be colored a different color and the appropriate parts should be labeled. This chapter has two sections of drawings, foot and ankle, and tibia, fibula and knee, which can be assigned separately or together.

▶ ANSWER KEY FOR STUDY QUESTIONS

1. 30
2. Dorsum pedis (dorsum); plantar
3. 14; miniature long bones
4. Hallux
5. Distal
6. Heads
7. 5th
8. Phalanges; tarsals
9. The metatarsals have to be much stronger as they support the weight of the body when a person is upright.
10. 7; short
11. Medial
12. Navicular
13. 4th and 5th
14. Calcaneus
15. Talus
16. Scaphoid
17. Calcaneus and os calcis
18. Calcaneus, navicular, tibia, and fibula
19. Talus
20. Pes planus is commonly called flatfoot. It occurs when the ligaments and tendons of the longitudinal arches are excessively strained and weakened.
21. Tibia and fibula; only the tibia is weight-bearing
22. 3; talus
23. Sustentaculum tali
24. The arches act like springs to cushion shocks when a person is applying weight to the foot.
25. Tibia
26. Trochlea
27. Anterior crest
28. Lateral malleolus; fibula
29. These large articular processes are located on the medial and lateral aspect of the proximal tibia.
30. This area is located on the superior surface of the tibial condyles. It is smooth and concave to articulate with the rounded condyles of the femur.
31. Base; fibular notch
32. Tibial tuberosity
33. Proximal
34. Femur
35. Intercondylar eminence or tibial spine
36. Apex or styloid process

37. Tibia and femur
38. Fibula
39. The fibular notch is a smooth articular surface on the posterolateral aspect of the lateral condyle of the tibia.
40. A tri-malleolar fracture
41. Medial and lateral condyles
42. On the anterior surface of the proximal tibia just inferior to the condyles
43. The epicondyles of the femur are prominences found on the superior portion of the medial and lateral condyles.
44. Intercondylar fossa
45. Anteriorly; laterally
46. Linea aspera
47. Fovea capitis
48. Fabella
49. The medial condyle
50. Ball and socket
51. Femoral neck
52. Patella
53. Greater; lesser
54. Intertrochanteric crest
55. Base; apex
56. Distal tibiofibular joint
57. Medial
58. The mortise or ankle joint is a three-sided joint formed by the talus and malleoli of the tibia and fibula. To demonstrate this joint radiographically, the lower limb must be internally rotated 15°.
59. Syndesmosis (fibrous joint)
60. Menisci
61. As a hinge joint, it allows flexion and extension; however, it also permits some rotational movement when the knee is flexed.
62. The area behind the knee
63. The cruciate ligaments extend between the femoral condyles and tibial plateau and cross for support and stability; the collateral ligaments bind the femur and tibia together medially and laterally.
64. G
65. G
66. H
67. H
68. C
69. Because the shoes can elevate the leg from the table and increase OID of the part
70. To demonstrate degenerative arthritis
71. Clubfoot
72. 10° cephalad
73. The 2nd metatarsophalangeal joint
74. 30°
75. Metatarsophalangeal sesamoid bones (a tangential projection was described)
76. Medial oblique
77. Lateral
78. 40° cephalad
79. 1–1½ in. distal to the medial malleolus
80. The tuberosity
81. To open the tibiotalar joint
82. Stress views of the ankle
83. The ankle joint is approximately ½ in. above the tip of the lateral malleolus.
84. 60–65 kVp; screen technique since the average measurement of the lower leg is less than 10 cm and a grid is not needed

85. The shaft of the tibia is more anterior than the fibula and only the proximal and distal aspects are superimposed.
86. AP projection
87. Lateral
88. 5° cephalad; it is necessary to open the tibiofemoral joint space
89. 45°
90. Lateral (external) oblique
91. 5° cephalad; to place the CR perpendicular to the joint space and prevent the medial condyle from superimposing the joint
92. AP and lateral
93. 20–30°
94. Lateral .
95. Perpendicular
96. 5–10°
97. Either the Camp–Coventry or Beclere Method can be used. Camp–Coventry: patient is prone, knee flexed approx. 40°, CR directed perpendicular to tibia at 40° angle; Beclere: patient is supine, knee is flexed so there is approx. 120° angle between femur and lower leg, CR directed at cephalic angle that is perpendicular to tibia
98. To rule out a horizontal (transverse) fracture
99. Approximately 10° cephalic or more to place the CR perpendicular to the joint space
100. The joint nearest the injury should be included with the shaft on a 14 × 17 in. film. The other joint can be radiographed on a smaller (10 × 12 in.) film.
101. To place the femur in a true AP position with the condyles symmetrical
102. The right leg will be brought forward over the leg of interest.
103. It is a bone length study that is usually performed bilaterally to illustrate a discrepancy in the length of the lower limbs.
104.

Projection	CR Angle/Angle of Part	Centering Point	Film Size	Structures Seen
Lateral foot	CR = perpendicular part = 90°	Tarsometatarsal joints	10 × 12 in. lw with axis of foot	Entire foot, particularly calcaneus, talus and navicular, superimposed metatarsals, phalanges, cuneiforms, and distal fibula and tibia
Medial (internal) oblique knee	CR = either perpendicular or 5° cephalad part = 45°	Knee joint (point just distal to apex of patella)	10 × 12 in. lw or 8 × 10 in. lw	Proximal tibiofibular articulation; also patella projected ⅓ to½ over medial femoral condyle; lateral femoral and tibial condyles well demonstrated
PA patella	CR = perpendicular part = leg rotated 5–10°	Midpoint of patella through popliteal region	8 × 10 in. lw	Entire patella superimposed over distal femur

Projection	CR Angle/Angle of Part	Centering Point	Film Size	Structures Seen
PA axial intercondylar fossa (Camp–Coventry Method)	CR = perpendicular to long axis of tibia part = knee flexed at 40–50° (if leg forms a 40° angle with table, then CR should be directed 40° caudally)	Popliteal depression	8 × 10 in. lw	Intercondylar fossa should be demonstrated, along with tibial plateaus, intercondylar eminence, medial and lateral femoral condyles, medial and lateral tibial condyles, distal shaft of the femur, and proximal shafts of the tibia and fibula.
AP femur	CR = perpendicular part = 0°	Either proximal or distal to midshaft, depending upon which joint will be included on the film	14 × 17 in. lw or 7×17 in. lw	Distal: femoral condyles superimposed, shaft of femur Proximal: greater trochanter superimposed over femoral neck, lesser trochanter in profile, femoral head in acetabulum of pelvis

DISCUSSION OF ATYPICAL CASE STUDIES ◄

1. The child's shoe and the board attached to the bottom of his foot would leave a definite artifact on the film. The rubberized sole would make visualization of the foot more difficult, and it may be hard to differentiate soft tissue, detailed anatomy, or subtle pathology. The actual rubberized treads may also be visible. As the nail is a foreign body, no angle would be used on the AP foot. It may be necessary to angle the tube if the child cannot flatten the foot, but the CR should be perpendicular to the foot. Obviously the radiograph would be taken before the board and nail were removed to establish the location of the nail and the amount of injury to the foot.

2. Since the woman cannot bend her knee due to severe rheumatoid arthritis, the plantar surface of her foot would be at an angle to the table. The cassette could be propped up under the foot so the plantar surface was flat on the surface. This process could be used for both the AP and medial oblique foot. For the AP foot the angulation of the CR would depend on the angle of the foot. The CR should be perpendicular to the longitudinal arch. These radiographs could also be accomplished with the woman standing on the cassette. The lateral would not pose a problem and could be done in the usual manner.

3. The hiker's leg could be placed diagonally on a 14 × 17 in. cassette. If both joints appear to fit on the cassette, it is important to increase the distance so neither joint will be collimated off. If the distance cannot be increased, the collimator should be opened in alignment with the 14 × 17 in. cassette, and the corners covered with lead strips to avoid excess scatter. If the leg will not fit on a 14 × 17 in. cassette diagonally, a 17 × 36 in. cassette could be used. If a sufficient SID cannot be obtained with the patient on the table, you could position him on the floor. The air splint should not be removed even though it may cause an artifact where the seam is joined and the plug may be visible on the radiograph.

4. The woman who has been hit on the knee by a log has probably fractured and/or dislocated her patella. The best projection for visualization of the patella is PA. This may be difficult to accomplish, however, as this may be very painful for the patient. The lateral and tangential patella would also be useful diagnostic radiographs. Her leg should not be straightened to facilitate the examination.

5. The developmentally disabled teenager should be radiographed while positioned on his side if possible. The AP could be accomplished by turning the patient into the supine positioning and straightening and immobilizing the knee. The lateral, intercondylar fossa and tangential patella projections can all be accomplished with the patient in the lateral position. The CR would be horizontal for the intercondylar fossa and tangential patella projections. The CR would be perpendicular to the lower leg for the intercondylar fossa radiograph. For the tangential patella, the CR should be directed to the femoropatellar joint space.

6. The cervical spine radiographs should be taken first on the man who fell off the roof. The entire regime of radiographs most likely will be performed while the patient remains in the supine position. The AP and lateral distal femur will be performed after the spine radiographs. The lateral femur would be done as a cross-table lateral. It would be important for two projections to be 90° apart as the radiographs were ordered for localization of the nail.

PELVIC GIRDLE 8

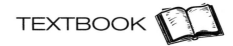

TEXTBOOK

Objectives

Following the completion of this chapter, the student will be able to:

1. Given diagrams, radiographs, or dry bones, name and describe the bones of the pelvic girdle, to include the ilium, ischium, pubis, sacrum, coccyx, and proximal femur.
2. Describe the locations and relationships of specific structures and positioning landmarks of the pelvic girdle (ie, ischial tuberosity is posterior and 1½ in. inferior to symphysis pubis).
3. Differentiate between the true and false divisions of the pelvis, to include structures and function.
4. Identify the structural differences on a male pelvis vs. a female pelvis, and differentiate between the sexes on radiographs of the pelvis.
5. Classify the articulations of the pelvic girdle and identify their type of movement.
6. Describe patient preparation and care relative to radiographic examination of the pelvic girdle.
7. List and describe the basic projections of the pelvic girdle, to include preferred type and size of image receptor, central ray location, and structures best visualized.
8. Practice positioning the basic projections of the pelvic girdle on another student or phantom.
9. Discuss the specific reason(s) for inverting the feet 15–20° during radiography of the pelvis and hip.
10. Describe procedural modifications for patients suspected of having a hip fracture.
11. Describe the breathing instructions for radiographic examinations of the pelvic girdle.
12. State the criteria used to determine positioning accuracy on radiographs of the pelvic girdle.
13. Evaluate radiographs of the pelvic girdle in terms of positioning, centering, image quality, radiographic anatomy, and pathology.
14. Describe equipment considerations and exposure factors relative to radiography of the pelvic girdle.
15. Define terminology associated with the pelvic girdle, to include anatomy, procedures, and pathology.

Chapter Outline

I. ANATOMY OF THE PELVIC GIRDLE

   A. Os Coxae

      1. ilium

      2. ischium

      3. pubis

      4. acetabulum

    B. Bony Pelvis
      1. false/greater pelvis
      2. true/lesser pelvis
      3. pelvic brim
      4. pelvic outlet
    C. Differences between Male and Female Pelves

II. ARTHROLOGY OF THE PELVIC GIRDLE
    A. Sacroiliac
    B. Coxal (hip)
    C. Symphysis Pubis
    D. Acetabulum

III. PROCEDURAL CONSIDERATIONS
    A. Patient Preparations
    B. Positioning Considerations
    C. Alternate Projections
    D. Pediatric Radiography
    E. Breathing Instructions
    F. Equipment Considerations
    G. Exposure Factors

IV. RADIOGRAPHIC POSITIONING OF THE PELVIC GIRDLE
    A. Pelvis: AP
      1. technical considerations
      2. shielding
      3. patient positioning
      4. part positioning
      5. central ray
      6. breathing instructions
      7. image evaluation
      8. critical anatomy
    B. Hip: AP, AP Oblique "Frog-leg," Lateral, Transfemoral "Cross-table" Lateral
      1. technical considerations
      2. shielding
      3. patient positioning
      4. part positioning
      5. central ray
      6. breathing instructions
      7. image evaluation
      8. critical anatomy
    C. Sacroiliac Joints: AP Oblique, PA Axial
      1. technical considerations
      2. shielding
      3. patient positioning
      4. part positioning
      5. central ray
      6. breathing instructions
      7. image evaluation
      8. critical anatomy

D. Anterior Pelvic Bones: AP Axial, Superoinferior Axial
 1. technical considerations
 2. shielding
 3. patient positioning
 4. part positioning
 5. central ray
 6. breathing instructions
 7. image evaluation
 8. critical anatomy
E. Acetabulum: AP Oblique, PA Axial Oblique
 1. technical considerations
 2. shielding
 3. patient positioning
 4. part positioning
 5. central ray
 6. breathing instructions
 7. image evaluation
 8. critical anatomy

V. SUMMARY
VI. CRITICAL THINKING & APPLICATION QUESTIONS
VII. FILM CRITIQUE

SAMPLE 50-MINUTE LESSON ◄

PREPARATION STEP

ESTIMATED TIME—10 MINUTES

A. Assemble teaching aids
 1. Overhead projector
 2. Overhead transparencies
  a. included in *Instructor's Resource Manual*
  b. trace drawings from *Applications Manual* on clear radiographic film
 3. Skeleton, disconnected pelvis
 4. Radiographs
B. Introduce topic of anatomy of the pelvic girdle. Lecture will include Chapter Objectives 1 and 2.
C. Opening discussion
 1. Review anatomy of the proximal femur.
 2. The pelvis has many parts that are named, which makes this chapter seem complicated. It is important to learn all the parts well.
 3. You must learn the anatomy well so you can visualize what anatomy is seen in each position that will be learned. Doing the drawings in the workbook will facilitate and reinforce this learning.

PRESENTATION STEP

ESTIMATED TIME—40 MINUTES

TEACHING OUTLINE	TEACHING AIDS & METHODS
I. Pelvic Girdle	*Pelvis transparency*
A. Formed by Paired Hip Bones (Ossa Coxae) and the Sacrum	

B. Supports Visceral Organs of Lower Abdomen
C. Functions to Attach Lower Limbs to Trunk
II. Anatomy of the Pelvic Girdle   *Radiograph of pelvis*
   A. Ossa Coxae/Innominate Bones/Hip Bones
      1. acetabulum   *Point out on pelvis*
         a. deep cup-shaped depression
         b. located on lower lateral margin of pelvis
         c. formed by bodies of
            (1) ilium—$\frac{2}{5}$
            (2) ischium—$\frac{2}{5}$
            (3) pubis—$\frac{1}{5}$
         d. bodies fuse together during late adolescence
            (18–20 yr)
      2. ilium
         a. ala
            (1) wings of ilium
            (2) project superiorly from body of ilium
            (3) upper curved portion is iliac crest   *Be sure students understand how*
               (a) extends from ASIS to PSIS   *iliac spines are named and their*
            (4) anterior portion   *location*
               (a) extends from ASIS to AIIS
            (5) posterior portion
               (a) extends from PSIS to PIIS
            (6) greater sciatic notch
               (a) extends from PIIS to ischial spine
                  (i) sciatic nerve passes through as
                      travels to leg
         b. body
            (1) forms inferior portion of ilium
            (2) forms upper $\frac{2}{5}$ of acetabulum
      3. ischium
         a. body
            (1) ischial spine
               (a) projects posteriorly from acetabulum
                   and medially into pelvic cavity
               (b) lesser sciatic notch just inferior to
                   spine
            (2) ischial tuberosity
               (a) process on posteroinferior aspect of
                   body
            (3) forms lower, posterior $\frac{2}{5}$ of acetabulum
         b. ramus
            (1) projects anteriorly, superiorly, and
                medially from ischial tuberosity to join
                inferior ramus of pubis
      4. pubis
         a. body
            (1) forms anterior $\frac{1}{5}$ of acetabulum
         b. rami
            (1) superior ramus
               (a) projects anteriorly and medially from
                   acetabulum
               (b) right and left superior rami form
                   symphysis pubis

          (2) inferior ramus
             (a) projects inferiorly and laterally from superior ramus
             (b) right and left inferior rami form pubic arch
    5. obturator foramen
       a. large opening on inferior aspect of hip bone
       b. formed by rami of ischium and pubis and body of ischium

APPLICATION STEP

ESTIMATED TIME—2 HOURS

Study Assignment

A. Begin reading Chapter 8 in the text.
B. Find all the anatomy discussed on the skeleton.
C. Find all the anatomy discussed on the radiographs of the pelvic girdle.
D. Begin Chapter 8 in the *Applications Manual.*

TESTING STEP

Questions on this material will be included in exam given at end of this chapter.

EXAM QUESTIONS ◄

Multiple Choice

1. What type of radiograph would the physician order if the patient has a possible acetabulum fracture?
   A. AP axial anterior pelvic bones
   B. superoinferior axial anterior pelvic bones
   C. AP pelvis
   D. AP oblique pelvis (Judet)

2. Which bony structure indicates the inferior portion of a correctly displayed transfemoral lateral hip radiograph?
   A. ischial spine
   B. ischial tuberosity
   C. acetabulum
   D. ASIS

3. What is the purpose of internally rotating the patient's legs 15–20° before making an exposure of the pelvis?
   A. to demonstrate the greater trochanter in profile
   B. to superimpose the lesser trochanter
   C. to demonstrate the femoral necks without foreshortening
   D. to better visualize the acetabulum

4. In which pelvis does the pelvic arch form an obtuse angle (greater than 90°)?
   A. male
   B. female

5. Which position/projection is requested to better visualize a possible rami fracture or to evaluate the pelvic outlet?
   A. AP axial anterior pelvic bones
   B. superoinferior axial anterior pelvic bones
   C. AP pelvis
   D. AP oblique pelvis (Judet)

6. The protocol for an AP pelvis states to internally rotate the legs. Under what condition would this directive NOT be followed?
   A. if a fractured hip is suspected
   B. if the patient has degenerative arthritis of the hip
   C. if there is evidence of an unusually long hip prosthesis
   D. if the patient is uncooperative

7. How is the grid cassette placed when performing a transfemoral lateral hip?
   A. lateral to the affected side, parallel to the shaft of the femur
   B. lateral to the affected side, parallel to the neck of the femur
   C. medial to the affected side, parallel to the greater trochanter
   D. medial to the affected side, parallel to the lesser trochanter

8. The patient is rotated 25–30° into an RPO position. The CR is centered 1 in. medial to the elevated ASIS. What structure will be best demonstrated on the radiograph?
   A. right acetabulum
   B. left acetabulum
   C. right SI joint
   D. left SI joint

9. Which oblique of the pelvis would BEST demonstrate the right obturator foramen?
   A. RPO
   B. LPO
   C. RAO
   D. LAO

10. For which position/projection is the patient instructed to flex the hip and knee of the affected side, rest the foot near the opposite side knee, and abduct the flexed leg 40°?
    A. AP oblique (frog-leg) lateral hip
    B. transfemoral (cross-table) lateral hip
    C. AP pelvis
    D. AP oblique SI joints

Matching

11. _____ Acetabulum
12. _____ Ossa coxae
13. _____ Right and left inferior rami
14. _____ SI joint

A. process on posteroinferior aspect of body of ischium
B. between sacrum and ilium
C. hip bones

15. _____ Right and left superior rami   D. forms pubic arch

E. posterior, superior iliac spine

F. receives the head of the femur

G. forms symphysis pubis

Answer Key

1. D	4. B	7. B	10. A	13. D
2. B	5. A	8. D	11. F	14. B
3. C	6. A	9. C	12. C	15. G

APPLICATIONS MANUAL

DRAWINGS ◄

The same directions apply to the drawings in this unit. Each bone should be colored a different color and the appropriate parts should be labeled. The femur drawings represent one of several ways to ensure that the entire femur is included on the AP and lateral femur.

ANSWER KEY FOR STUDY QUESTIONS ◄

1. Ossa coxae or innominate bones
2. Ilium, ischium, and pubis
3. A. support the visceral organs of the lower abdomen and B. attach the lower limb to the trunk of the body
4. Acetabulum
5. Ischium
6. Ilium
7. Pubis
8. Acetabulum
9. Pubis
10. Ala
11. It is the slightly concave inner surface of the ala of the ilium.
12. Anterior superior iliac spine (ASIS)
13. Greater sciatic notch
14. Iliac crest
15. The body is the inferior aspect of the ilium forming the upper part of the acetabulum.
16. The ischium
17. Auricular surface
18. Ischial tuberosity
19. Ramus
20. Posterior
21. ⅖
22. ⅖
23. ⅕
24. Superior rami
25. Inferior ramus

26. Obturator foramen
27. The pubic arch is the inverted V-shaped area formed by the inferior rami of the right and left pubic bones.
28. Ischial spine
29. Pubic crest
30. Medially
31. False
32. Upper margin of the symphysis pubis; sacral promontory
33. At the lower border of the greater sciatic notch
34. Pelvic inlet
35. True
36. Pubic arch; coccyx; ischial spines and tuberosities
37. False
38. Lesser; greater
39. Female
40. The pubic arch is obtuse or greater than 90° on a female pelvis and more acute or less than 90° on a male pelvis
41. Ultrasound
42. Acetabulum and head of the femur
43. Coxal refers to the hip joint
44. The sacroiliac (SI) joints
45. Cartilaginous; amphiarthrodial
46. In a child, cartilage is present between the articulations (synchondrosis) of the ilium, ischium, and pubis at the acetabulum, but as the child ages, the bones fuse solidly together (synostosis).
47. Synovial
48. Diarthrodial with ball and socket movement
49. The upper part of the joint is amphiarthrodial, but the lower portion is diarthrodial with gliding movement.
50. Also called avascular necrosis, it is an idiopathic condition caused by loss of the blood supply to the femoral head, resulting in abnormal growth and bone necrosis.
51. To find out if the patient has a prosthesis, and if so, how long it is so that it can be included in its entirety on the radiograph
52. To overcome the curvature of the femurs and place the proximal femurs in a true AP position
53. Rotation of the leg can cause severe pain and also vascular damage, which could lead to the formation of a blood clot.
54. When the legs are correctly rotated 15–20° internally, the lesser trochanters will not be seen or may be minimally seen on the medial aspect of the proximal femurs.
55. Draw an imaginary line between the ASIS and symphysis pubis; bisect the line and extend a line perpendicular to the bisection. The femoral neck is approximately 2½ in. distal to the point of bisection. An alternate method is to localize the point 2 in. medial and inferior to the ASIS over the inguinal crease.
56. Since a fracture is suspected, the patient should not abduct his/her leg. Therefore, the transfemoral (surgical) lateral projection should be obtained.
57. Because the joints are positioned obliqued in the body
58. 25–30°
59. Left
60. 30–35° caudad
61. Asymmetry of the size and shape of the ala of the ilia and the obturator foramina
62. 40°
63. Approximately ⅓ of the proximal femur should be included; if a prosthesis is present, it should be included in its entirety.
64. Perpendicular
65. Take an AP axial projection with the patient on her back and the central ray angled 30–35° cephalad

66. 30–35° cephalad; 20–35° cephalad. The female pelvis is generally more shallow than the male pelvis and therefore the angulation must be increased to separate the rami of the ischium and pubis.
67. The superior and inferior pubic rami are superimposed medially, while the superior pubic rami and ischial rami are almost superimposed laterally.
68. 45°
69. 12° caudad; coccyx
70. True
71. False; only the ischium and pubis encircle the obturator foramen.
72. False; the sacrum is generally short, broad, and less curved on the female pelvis.
73. True
74. True
75.

Projection	CR Angle/ Angle of Part	Centering Point	Film Size	Structures Seen
AP pelvis	CR = perpendicular part = 0°	Approximately 2 in. above symphysis pubis (lower if hips are area of interest)	14 × 17 in cw	Entire pelvis—iliac crests, ala, ASISs, ischial and pubic rami, symphysis pubis, ischial tuberosities, acetabula, femoral heads, and greater trochanters
AP oblique (frog-leg) hip (mod. Cleaves)	CR = perpendicular part = leg abducted 40°	The femoral neck	10 × 12 in. lw or cw	Acetabulum, femoral head, femoral neck without foreshortening, greater and lesser trochanters superimposed
Lateral hip (Lauenstein method)	CR = perpendicular part = approx. 90° to body	The hip joint	10 × 12 in. cw or lw	Acetabulum, femoral head, femoral neck, greater and lesser trochanters partially superimposed over femoral neck and femoral shaft, respectively
LPO for SI joints	CR = perpendicular part = side of interest is elevated 25–30°	1 in. medial to ASIS on side of interest	8 × 10 in. lw	Right sacroiliac joint open
AP oblique acetabulum (Judet method)	CR = perpendicular part = side of interest elevated 45°	Femoral head	10 × 12 in. lw	Acetabulum and femoral head

DISCUSSION OF ATYPICAL CASE STUDIES ◄

1. The woman who was struck by a bicycle and presents with her left foot turned outward and left leg bent appears to be exhibiting the classic signs of a left hip fracture. The AP hip or pelvis would not pose a problem if she were carefully transported from the stretcher to the radiographic table. Obviously her left leg should not be manipulated in any way before taking the radiograph. The lateral hip would be obtained by doing a transfemoral (cross-table) lateral. Again, no manipulation of the injured leg is indicated.

2. The tall 20-year-old male involved in the motorcycle accident would require several radiographs to visualize his entire femur. The two projections of the hip would be an AP and transfemoral (cross-table) lateral. His leg should not be manipulated for either radiograph. Several 14 × 17 in. films would be used for imaging the remaining femur as this patient is tall. The lateral would be performed as a cross-table.

3. Oblique radiographs of the SI joints could certainly be obtained using anterior oblique positions rather than posterior oblique positions when the patient is unable to lie supine on the table. The right SI joint would be obtained by turning the patient in the RAO position and the left SI joint would be obtained by turning the patient into the LAO position. The cephalic angulation of the CR is used when obtaining AP axial SI joints so the modification would be to use a caudal angle of the CR if it is necessary to do the axial SI joints with the patient prone.

BONY THORAX 9

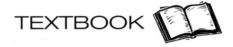

Objectives

Following the completion of this chapter, the student will be able to:

1. Given diagrams, radiographs, or dry bones, name and describe the bones of the bony thorax, to include the ribs and sternum.
2. Identify any surface markings found on the bones of the bony thorax.
3. List any additional names for the structures of the bony thorax, particularly the sternum.
4. Classify the articulations of the bony thorax and identify their type of movement, if applicable.
5. List and describe the basic projections of the bony thorax, to include preferred type and size of image receptor, central ray location, and structures best visualized.
6. Practice positioning the basic projections of the bony thorax on another student or phantom.
7. State the criteria used to determine positioning accuracy on radiographs of the bony thorax.
8. Discuss the recommended breathing instructions for radiographic examinations of the bony thorax.
9. Evaluate radiographs of the bony thorax in terms of positioning, centering, image quality, radiographic anatomy, and pathology.
10. Describe equipment considerations and exposure factors relative to radiography of the bony thorax.
11. Define terminology associated with the bony thorax, to include anatomy, procedures, and pathology.

Chapter Outline

I. ANATOMY OF THE BONY THORAX
   A. Sternum
   B. Ribs
II. ARTHROLOGY OF THE BONY THORAX
   A. Sternoclavicular
   B. Manubriosternal
   C. Xiphisternal
   D. Sternocostal
      1. 1st pair
      2. 2nd–7th pair
   E. Costochondral
   F. Interchondral

G. Costovertebral

H. Costotransverse

III. PROCEDURAL CONSIDERATIONS

A. Patient Preparations

B. Positioning Considerations

C. Breathing Instructions

D. Equipment Considerations

E. Exposure Factors

IV. RADIOGRAPHIC POSITIONING OF THE BONY THORAX

A. Ribs: AP (Above and Below Diaphragm), AP Oblique

1. technical considerations

2. shielding

3. patient positioning

4. part positioning

5. central ray

6. breathing instructions

7. image evaluation

8. critical anatomy

B. Sternum: RAO, Lateral

1. technical considerations

2. shielding

3. patient positioning

4. part positioning

5. central ray

6. breathing instructions

7. image evaluation

8. critical anatomy

C. Sternoclavicular Joints: PA Oblique

1. technical considerations

2. shielding

3. patient positioning

4. part positioning

5. central ray

6. breathing instructions

7. image evaluation

8. critical anatomy

V. SUMMARY

VI. CRITICAL THINKING & APPLICATION QUESTIONS

VII. FILM CRITIQUE

SAMPLE 50-MINUTE LESSON ◄

PREPARATION STEP	ESTIMATED TIME—10 MINUTES

A. Assemble teaching aids
   1. Overhead projector
   2. Overhead transparencies
       a. included in *Instructor's Resource Manual*
       b. trace drawings from *Applications Manual* on clear radiographic film
   3. Skeleton
   4. Radiographs
B. Introduce topic of articulations and procedural considerations of the bony thorax. Lecture will include Chapter Objectives 4 and 5.
C. Opening discussion
   1. The basic anatomy was discussed during the last class. We will be continuing with the objectives beginning with articulations of the bony thorax. We will then continue with procedural considerations for positioning of this area.
   2. Obtaining optimal radiographs of the ribs and sternum can be very challenging and frustrating. It is very important to learn the anatomy well, and practice positioning so these exams don't seem so overwhelming when they are requested.

PRESENTATION STEP	ESTIMATED TIME—40 MINUTES

TEACHING OUTLINE	TEACHING AIDS & METHODS
I. Arthrology of the Bony Thorax	*Transparency of joints*

I. Arthrology of the Bony Thorax
   A. Sternoclavicular Joint
       1. synovial joint
       2. diarthrodial gliding
       3. where clavicle articulates with axial skeleton
   B. Manubriosternal Joint
       1. cartilaginous joint
       2. synchondrosis/synostosis joint
       3. amphiarthrodial/synarthrodial
       4. slightly movable synchondrosis joint until ossifies and becomes immovable synostosis joint
   C. Xiphisternal joint
       1. same structure as manubriosternal joint
       2. ossifies around age 40
           a. synarthrodial immovable joint
   D. Sternocostal joint
       1. 1st pair
           a. synchondrosis
           b. synarthrodial immovable
       2. 2nd–7th pair
           a. synovial
           b. diarthrodial gliding
   E. Costochondral
       1. synchondrosis
       2. synarthrodial immovable
   F. Interchondral
       1. synovial
       2. diarthrodial gliding

G. Costovertebral
   1. synovial
   2. diarthrodial gliding
H. Costotransverse
   1. synovial
   2. diarthrodial gliding
II. Procedural Considerations
  A. Patient Preparation
    1. first check to be sure correct patient
    2. have patient remove all clothing and jewelry from between the neck and hips and put on a patient gown
    3. pertinent patient history is necessary to determine which projections to perform and the breathing instructions to be used
  B. Positioning Considerations
    1. ribs
      a. chest radiograph often included in protocol
        (1) expiration
      b. an upright exam will often be more comfortable for the patient
      c. ribs above diaphragm
        (1) upright
      d. ribs below diaphragm
        (1) recumbent
      e. rib protocol varies and depends on the site of injury
        (1) AP/PA   *Radiographic examples*
        (2) oblique of area of interest
          (a) rotate to place area of interest roughly parallel to film
    2. sternum
      a. must rotate patient so sternum will not be superimposed on spine
      b. RAO position also projects sternum over homogeneous heart shadow   *Rotate skeleton into RAO position while placing fist inside thorax to represent heart*
      c. rotate patient 15–20°
        (1) thinner patient—20°
        (2) larger patient—15°
      d. lateral sternum should be done upright and at 72 in. SID when possible
    3. SC joints
      a. RAO/LAO   *Demonstrate how SC joint moves to up side of spine on RAO skeleton*
        (1) patient rotated 10–15°
        (2) demonstrates side down although actual joint will be across the spine toward the up side
  C. Breathing Instructions
    1. upper ribs—deep inspiration
    2. lower ribs—full expiration
    3. RAO sternum—breathing technique full expiration
    4. Lateral sternum—full inspiration
    5. SC joints—expiration

D. Equipment Consideration
  1. a grid is recommended for most radiography of
     the bony thorax
  2. lateral sternum
     a. can do without grid due to air gap
     b. 72 in. SID to minimize magnification
  3. RAO sternum
     a. can reduce distance to 30 in.
        (1) increases blurring of ribs and lung detail
E. Exposure Factors
  1. upper ribs and RAO sternum
     a. 60–65 kVp
  2. lower ribs
     a. 65–70 kVp
  3. lateral sternum
     a. 70–80 kVp

APPLICATION STEP   ESTIMATED TIME—2 HOURS

Study Assignment

A. Continue reading Chapter 9 in the text.
B. Continue Chapter 9 in the *Applications Manual.*
C. Be sure you can locate all the anatomy discussed on a skeleton and on a radiograph.

TESTING STEP

Questions on this material will be included in exam given at end of this chapter.

EXAM QUESTIONS ◄

Matching

1. _____ Manubrium   A. at level of T3–4

2. _____ Gladiolus   B. located at posterior end of rib

3. _____ Jugular notch   C. upper portion of sternum

4. _____ Sternal angle   D. at the level of T2–3

5. _____ Sternal extremity E. located at medial end of clavicle

                                F. at the level of C7–T1

                                G. body of sternum

Multiple Choice

6. Why is the sternum radiographed with the patient in an RAO position?
   A. so the sternum will not be superimposed by the heart
   B. so the sternum will not be superimposed by the spine
   C. this is the most comfortable position for the patient
   D. the patient is better able to take in a deep breath while in this position

7. When the patient is positioned in an LAO position to visualize the left SC joint, the left SC joint is projected to the _____ of the vertebrae.
   A. left
   B. right

8. The normal rotation for an RAO sternum is 15–20°. What criteria should you use to decide how many degrees to rotate a specific patient?
   A. the female sternum requires a greater angulation than a male sternum
   B. the male sternum requires a greater angulation than a female sternum
   C. a broad chest requires less angulation than a thinner chest
   D. a thinner chest requires less angulation than a broad chest

9. How would you position a patient for oblique ribs if the injury were on the right anterior side?
   A. LAO
   B. RAO
   C. LPO
   D. RPO

10. How would you position a patient for oblique ribs if the injury were on the left posterior side?
    A. LAO
    B. RAO
    C. LPO
    D. RPO

11. Your patient's rib injury is approximately at the 6th rib. What are the appropriate breathing instructions for this patient?
    A. stop breathing
    B. keep breathing normally
    C. take in a deep breath, let it all the way out
    D. take in a deep breath and hold it

12. What are the appropriate breathing instructions when radiographing the sternum in the RAO position?
    A. no specific breathing instructions should be given so the patient breathes normally
    B. take in a deep breath, let it all the way out
    C. take in a deep breath and hold it
    D. stop breathing

Answer Key

1. C	4. A	7. B	10. C
2. G	5. E	8. C	11. D
3. D	6. B	9. A	12. A

APPLICATIONS MANUAL

DRAWINGS ◄

The same directions apply to the drawings in this unit. Each bone should be colored a different color and the appropriate parts should be labeled.

ANSWER KEY FOR STUDY QUESTIONS ◄

1. Sternum and 12 pairs of ribs
2. The sternum forms the anterior part of the cage and the ribs wrap around from front to back on both sides to articulate with the thoracic vertebrae, which form the posterior aspect of the cage.
3. Sternum
4. 12
5. Flat
6. Vertebral and sternal
7. Posterior
8. Tubercle
9. Angle
10. Costal groove
11. At the anterior end of the rib, attaching the rib to the sternum
12. The head
13. Intercostal
14. Sternal
15. Vertebrosternal
16. The 1st–7th pairs are true ribs because their costal cartilages attach directly to the sternum.
17. Vertebrochondral ribs
18. The lower five pairs (8th–12th)
19. The costal arch is the curved margin formed by the costal cartilage of the 1st–10th ribs on each side with the xiphoid process in between.
20. 11th and 12th
21. 2nd; 9th; 1st, 10th, 11th, and 12th
22. Because of the presence of the blood vessels and nerves running along the inner surface of the shaft of the rib
23. They elevate the ribs during breathing, which in turn increases the width of the chest and lung volume.
24. It is not demonstrated radiographically unless it is calcified.
25. Manubrium, body, and xiphoid process
26. Flat
27. Manubrium
28. Gladiolus
29. Xiphoid process
30. Sternal angle
31. Xiphoid process
32. The xiphoid process can break away from the sternal body and lacerate the heart and/or liver.
33. Rib; cartilage
34. The disk space (intervertebral joint) between T-3 and T-4
35. Ensiform process

36. Since the sternum is a flat bone, it is basically composed of cancellous bone. Red blood cells are produced in the red bone marrow occupying the trabeculae of the cancellous bone. The red bone marrow can be extracted from the sternum and transplanted intravenously into a recipient. The ilium of the pelvis is used more frequently for this purpose.
37. Jugular notch; suprasternal or manubrial notch
38. The disk space (intervertebral joint) between T-9 and T-10
39. The disk space (intervertebral joint) between T-2 and T-3
40. Manubrium
41. These slight depressions are located on the manubrium to either side of the jugular notch.
42. A small flattened or depressed articular surface
43. Sternoclavicular joint
44. 40
45. Manubriosternal
46. The 1st sternocostal joint is a synchondrosis, that is immovable; the 2nd–7th sternocostal joints are synovial and diarthrodial with gliding movement.
47. The sternal extremities of the ribs and their corresponding costal cartilages
48. Costovertebral; costotransverse
49. Synovial; diarthrodial with gliding movement
50. LPO or RAO
51. RPO or LAO
52. In an RAO position, the sternum is projected over the heart shadow, allowing for a more uniform density and better visualization.
53. 15–20°
54. Less
55. 10–15°
56. LAO
57. It allows the patient to breathe quietly, thus blurring the overlying lung markings and making the sternum more visible.
58. Deep expiration
59. Since the sternum is not touching the film on the lateral projection, the increased OID causes magnification. To minimize magnification, 72 in. is used.
60. The shorter SID increases the blurring effect of the posterior ribs and lung detail.
61. The upper 8–10 ribs should be demonstrated.
62. The lower 4–6 ribs should be demonstrated.
63. To provide high contrast between the ribs and lungs
64. T6–7
65. Rotate the patient more until the sternum is no longer superimposed over the spine.
66. Deep inspiration
67. Nearest
68. To pull the shoulders back so they do not superimpose the manubrium
69. To pull the scapulae away from the ribs
70. False; radiography of the ribs can be performed in either the recumbent or erect position.
71. True
72. True
73. False; the body of the sternum is the longest part of the bone.
74. True

75.

Projection	CR Angle/ Angle of Part	Centering Point	Film Size	Structures Seen
Lateral sternum	CR = horizontal part = 90°	Midpoint of sternum	10 × 12 in. lw	Manubrium, sternal angle, body, and xiphoid process should be demonstrated anterior to lung tissue.
RAO SC joints	CR = perpendicular part = 10–15°	Right SC joint at level of jugular notch	8 × 10 in. cw	Right sternoclavicular joint free of superimposition
RPO ribs	CR = perpendicular part = 45°	Adjust centering point, depending upon area of injury. Center to midpoint of cassette	14 × 17 in. lw	Axillary margin of right ribs and vertebral extremities of left ribs
AP ribs below the diaphragm	CR = perpendicular part = 0°	Center to midpoint of cassette—left border of cassette is approx. 1½ in. below the iliac crests	14 × 17 in. cw	Lower ribs 8–12 should be demonstrated in the abdomen.

DISCUSSION OF ATYPICAL CASE STUDIES

1. The sternum radiograph should be attempted with the patient in the LPO position as he cannot lie in a prone position due to his recent heart surgery. The lateral sternum can be accomplished using a horizontal beam, and the SID should be 72 in. if there is enough room. It may be necessary to do tomography of the sternum, however, as it may not be adequately imaged when the patient is in the LPO position rather than the standard RAO position.

2. An AP projection using a grid would not pose a problem with the patient shackled to the stretcher. The obliques would have to be LPO and RPO. It would not be possible to do a PA projection or anterior obliques on this patient. By doing an LPO of the thorax above and below the diaphragm, and an RPO of the thorax above and below the diaphragm, there should be enough information to diagnose possible rib fractures.

10 VERTEBRAL COLUMN

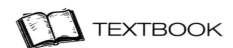 TEXTBOOK

Objectives

Following the completion of this chapter, the student will be able to:

1. Given diagrams, radiographs, or dry bones, name and describe the bones of the vertebral column.
2. Identify the topographic landmarks associated with specific vertebrae.
3. Differentiate between the curves of the vertebral column, to include primary curves, compensatory curves, lordosis, kyphosis, and scoliosis.
4. Describe the structural differences between the cervical, thoracic, and lumbar vertebrae.
5. Classify the articulations in the vertebral column according to structure and identify their type of movement, if applicable.
6. List and describe the basic projections of the vertebral column, to include preferred type and size of image receptor, central ray location, and structures best visualized.
7. Describe the procedural adaptations necessary for radiography of the spine in a trauma situation.
8. Identify and describe projections that can be used to evaluate mobility and abnormal lateral curvature of the spine.
9. Practice positioning the basic projections of the vertebral column on another student or phantom.
10. Describe equipment considerations and exposure factors relative to radiography of the vertebral column.
11. State the criteria used to determine positioning accuracy on radiographs of the vertebral column.
12. Evaluate radiographs of the vertebral column in terms of positioning, centering, image quality, radiographic anatomy, and pathology.
13. Define terminology associated with the vertebral column, to include anatomy, procedures, and pathology.

Chapter Outline

I. ANATOMY OF THE VERTEBRAL COLUMN
  A. Regional Divisions
    1. cervical
    2. thoracic
    3. lumbar
    4. sacrum
    5. coccyx
  B. Curvatures of the Spine
    1. primary curves
    2. secondary or compensatory curves

      3. kyphosis

      4. lordosis

      5. scoliosis

  C. Characteristics of the Typical Vertebra

      1. body

      2. vertebral arch

  D. Cervical Vertebrae

      1. articular pillar

      2. vertebral prominens

  E. Thoracic Vertebrae

      1. costal facets

  F. Lumbar Vertebrae

      1. pars interarticularis

  G. Sacrum

  H. Coccyx

II. ARTHROLOGY OF THE VERTEBRAL COLUMN

  A. Intervertebral

  B. Interarticular

      1. atlanto-occipital

      2. atlantoaxial

      3. zygapophyseal C2–S1

  C. Costovertebral

  D. Costotransverse

III. TOPOGRAPHIC LANDMARKS

IV. PROCEDURAL CONSIDERATIONS

  A. Patient Preparation

      1. cervical spine

      2. thoracic spine

      3. lumbosacral spine

      4. trauma care

  B. Positioning Considerations

  C. Trauma Considerations

      1. cervical spine lateral evaluation

  D. Alternate Projections

      1. hyperflexion/hyperextension studies

      2. scoliosis

  E. Breathing Instructions

  F. Exposure Factors

  G. Equipment Considerations

V. RADIOGRAPHIC POSITIONING OF THE SPINE

  A. Cervical Spine: AP, AP Atlas and Axis, AP Axial Oblique, Lateral, Hyperflexion/ Hyperextension Lateral, Swimmer's

      1. technical considerations

      2. shielding

      3. patient positioning

      4. part positioning

      5. central ray

    6. breathing instructions

    7. image evaluation

    8. critical anatomy

B. Thoracic Spine: AP, PA Oblique, Lateral

    1. technical considerations

    2. shielding

    3. patient positioning

    4. part positioning

    5. central ray

    6. breathing instructions

    7. image evaluation

    8. critical anatomy

C. Lumbar Spine: AP, AP Oblique, Lateral, Hyperflexion/Hyperextension Lateral

    1. technical considerations

    2. shielding

    3. patient positioning

    4. part positioning

    5. central ray

    6. breathing instructions

    7. image evaluation

    8. critical anatomy

D. Lumbosacral Junction: AP Axial, Lateral

    1. technical considerations

    2. shielding

    3. patient positioning

    4. part positioning

    5. central ray

    6. breathing instructions

    7. image evaluation

    8. critical anatomy

E. Sacrum: AP, Lateral

    1. technical considerations

    2. shielding

    3. patient positioning

    4. part positioning

    5. central ray

    6. breathing instructions

    7. image evaluation

    8. critical anatomy

F. Coccyx: AP, Lateral

    1. technical considerations

    2. shielding

    3. patient positioning

    4. part positioning

    5. central ray

    6. breathing instructions

        7. image evaluation

        8. critical anatomy

    G. Scoliosis Projection: PA, Lateral

        1. technical considerations

        2. shielding

        3. patient positioning

        4. part positioning

        5. central ray

        6. breathing instructions

        7. image evaluation

        8. critical anatomy

  VI. SUMMARY

  VII. CRITICAL THINKING & APPLICATION QUESTIONS

  VIII. FILM CRITIQUE

SAMPLE 50-MINUTE LESSON ◄

PREPARATION STEP   ESTIMATED TIME—10 MINUTES

A. Assemble teaching aids
    1. Overhead projector
    2. Overhead transparencies
       a. included in *Instructor's Resource Manual*
       b. trace drawings from *Applications Manual* on clear radiographic film
    3. Skeleton
    4. Radiographs
B. Introduce topic of positioning of the thoracic spine. Lecture will include Chapter Objectives 6, 10, and 11 as they relate to the thoracic spine.
C. Opening discussion
    1. Anatomy, procedural considerations, and positioning of the cervical spine have been presented. This lecture will continue with the positioning of the thoracic spine.
    2. Be sure you can visualize the anatomy that is visualized on each projection or position discussed.
    3. All children and adults of reproductive age should be shielded for radiographic exams of the thoracic and lumbar spine unless it obstructs necessary anatomy to be visualized. A grid is necessary for all exams of the thoracic and lumbar spine. The SID for the majority of thoracic and lumbar spine radiographs is 40 in., and any exceptions will be noted when the position/projection is covered.
    4. Most radiographic exams of the thoracic and lumbar spine should be done on expiration. Exceptions will also be noted when the position/projection is covered.

PRESENTATION STEP   ESTIMATED TIME—40 MINUTES

TEACHING OUTLINE	TEACHING AIDS & METHODS
I. Positioning of the Thoracic Spine	*Transparency of spine*
A. Lateral Cervicothoracic Spine (Swimmer's)	
1. technical considerations	*Swimmer's radiograph*
a. 10 × 12 in.	

2. positioning
    a. upright recumbent, or cross-table
    b. patient in true lateral position with arm
       nearest the film raised and shoulder moved
       slightly anterior
    c. other shoulder depressed and moved slightly
       posterior
    d. thoracic spine must remain lateral
3. central ray
    a. perpendicular to T-1 if shoulders separated
       appropriately
    b. 3–5° caudad angle to T-1
       (1) helps separate humeral heads if necessary
4. structures visualized
    a. bony and soft tissue structures of
    b. the neck and C-5 through T-4
    c. intervertebral disk spaces and vertebral bodies   *Demonstrate how difficult it can be*
       of C-4 through T-4   *to count vertebrae when C-1 not*
    d. must include C-1 in many trauma clinical sites   *included*
       to facilitate counting of vertebrae
B. AP Thoracic Spine
    1. technical considerations   *T spine radiographs*
        a. 14 × 17 in. or 7 × 17 in.
    2. positioning
        a. supine on table
        b. patient's head on anode side of tube   *Explain "anode-heel" effect*
           (1) utilizes the "anode-heel" effect   *anode+/←cathode-*
    3. central ray
        a. perpendicular to T-1
        b. center to cassette placed with top edge
           1½–2 in. above shoulders
    4. structures visualized
        a. intervertebral disk spaces and vertebral bodies
           of C-1 through L-1
    5. NOTE: some sites use wedge filter or IV bag
             over T spine to achieve more even density
             on radiograph
C. PA Oblique Thoracic Spine
    1. technical considerations   *T spine radiographs*
    2. positioning
        a. upright, recumbent
        b. from lateral position rotate patient 20° toward
           the film
        c. both sides are done for comparison
           (1) RAO and LAO
           (2) RPO and LPO sometimes done in place
               of anterior obliques
    3. central ray
        a. perpendicular to T-7
        b. center to cassette placed with top edge
           1½–2 in. above shoulders
    4. structures visualized
        a. anterior obliques—zygapophyseal joints
           nearest the table or upright Bucky

D. Lateral Thoracic Spine
   1. technical considerations   *T spine radiographs*
      a. 14×17 in. or 7×17 in.
   2. positioning
      a. upright or recumbent lateral
      b. midaxillary plane to midline of cassette
      c. T spine parallel to cassette
   3. central ray
      a. perpendicular to T-7
      b. parallel to intervertebral joints
         (1) may require cephalic angle
      c. center to cassette placed with top edge
         $1\frac{1}{2}$–2 in. above shoulders
   4. breathing instructions
      a. quiet breathing   *Explain term* breathing technique
         (1) low MA, high time
         (2) blurs out lung and rib detail
   5. structures visualized
      a. intervertebral foramina
      b. intervertebral disk spaces and vertebral bodies
         of T-3 through L-1

APPLICATION STEP   ESTIMATED TIME—2 HOURS

Study Assignment

A. Continue reading Chapter 10 in the text.
B. Continue Chapter 10 in the *Applications Manual.*
C. Compare the positioning drawings in the *Applications Manual* to a corresponding radiograph.
D. Critique radiographs for image quality and proper positioning. Be sure you can locate the anatomic parts listed on the drawing worksheets on each of the radiographs.

TESTING STEP

Questions on this material will be included in exam given at end of this chapter.

EXAM QUESTIONS ◄

Multiple Choice

1. The patient is in a 45° oblique LPO position. There is a 15° cephalic angle on the tube and the CR is centered to C-4. Which anatomic part is visualized?
   A. left zygapophyseal joint
   B. right zygapophyseal joint
   C. left intervertebral foramen
   D. right intervertebral foramen

2. The patient is in a 20° down from the lateral RAO position. The CR is perpendicular to the film through T-7. Which anatomic part is visualized?
   A. left zygapophyseal joint
   B. right zygapophyseal joint
   C. left intervertebral foramen
   D. right intervertebral foramen

3. The patient is in a 45° oblique LAO position. The CR is perpendicular to the film through L-3. Which anatomic part is visualized?
   A. left zygapophyseal joint
   B. right zygapophyseal joint
   C. left intervertebral foramen
   D. right intervertebral foramen

4. Which anatomic parts form the intervertebral foramina?
   A. superior and inferior vertebral notches
   B. superior and inferior articular processes
   C. anterior and posterior vertebral foramen
   D. anterior and posterior vertebral arch

5. Which anatomic parts form the zygapophyseal joints?
   A. superior and inferior vertebral notches
   B. superior and inferior articular processes
   C. anterior and posterior vertebral foramen
   D. anterior and posterior vertebral arch

6. The pars interarticularis is located
   A. between the zygapophyseal joints on the cervical spine
   B. between the zygapophyseal joints on the lumbar spine
   C. between the superior and inferior articular processes on the cervical spine
   D. between the superior and inferior articular processes on the lumbar spine

7. What condition occurs when there is a forward displacement of one lumbar vertebral body over the vertebra or sacrum beneath it?
   A. herniated disk
   B. degenerative joint disease
   C. spondylolisthesis
   D. rheumatoid arthritis

8. The first zygapophyseal joint of the vertebral column is located:
   A. between the superior articulating facets of C-1 and the condyles of the occipital bone
   B. between the inferior surface of the lateral masses of C-1 and the superior articular surface of C-2
   C. between the inferior articular surface of C-2 and the superior articular surface of C-3
   D. between the inferior articular process of L-5 and the superior surface of the sacrum

9. Which type of radiographs are ordered to evaluate the degree of *anteroposterior* mobility, ligament injuries, or potential instability of the cervical spine?
   A. hyperflexion and hyperextension
   B. AP and left lateral
   C. right and left lateral side-bending radiographs
   D. upright and supine left and right lateral radiographs

10. You are looking at an optimal radiograph of the lateral cervical spine. A grid was not used for this radiograph. How was it possible to obtain the radiograph without using a grid?

   A. a 72 in. SID was used

   B. the "anode-heel" effect was utilized

   C. the OID of the cervical spine causes an air gap to produce an effect similar to that of a grid

   D. the patient's shoulders were depressed sufficiently to visualize the cervical spine without the grid

11. What are the optimal breathing instructions to a cooperative patient to facilitate better visualization of the odontoid on a radiograph?

   A. breathe normally

   B. take in a deep breath and hold it

   C. take in a deep breath and blow it all the way out

   D. hold your mouth open and say "ah" during the exposure

Matching

From the column on the right, choose all answers that apply to each item in the column on the left.

12. _____ Cervical spine   A. kyphosis

13. _____ Thoracic spine   B. lordosis

14. _____ Lumbar spine   C. primary curve

15. _____ Sacrum   D. secondary curve

Answer Key

1. D	4. A	7. C	10. C	13. C, A
2. B	5. B	8. B	11. D	14. D, B
3. B	6. D	9. A	12. D, C	15. C, A

APPLICATIONS MANUAL

DRAWINGS ◄

Each section of the spine should be colored a different color. The oblique cervical and lumbar spine drawings are an excellent learning tool for the student to reinforce which parts are visualized on each section of the spine.

ANSWER KEY FOR STUDY QUESTIONS ◄

1. Cervical
Thoracic
Lumbar
Sacrum
Coccyx

2. 4

3. A child has approximately 33 bones because the sacral segments and coccygeal segments have not fused, while an adult averages 26 bones.

4. Thoracic and sacral
5. Cervical and lumbar
6. Compensatory refers to the secondary curves, which develop after birth; they curve in the opposite direction of the primary curves to help a person maintain an erect posture.
7. Cervical and lumbar
8. Thoracic and sacral
9. Kyphosis
10. Lordosis
11. Scoliosis
12. Body and vertebral arch
13. Vertebral arch
14. Irregular
15. Body
16. Cancellous
17. Pedicles
18. Vertebral
19. Intervertebral
20. Pedicles
21. Lamina
22. Right and left transverse processes; right and left superior articular processes; right and left inferior articular processes; spinous process
23. 45°
24. Spina bifida
25. The vertebral canal is formed by consecutive vertebral foramina when the vertebrae are stacked in a column.
26. Pedicle and lamina
27. Spinous processes
28. 15°
29. Spinous process
30. 7, 12, and 5
31. C-7; because its spinous process is very prominent and can be palpated at the back of the neck
32. Transverse processes
33. Bifid means forked or split. The spinous processes of C2–C7 have bifid tips.
34. On the vertebral arch directly posterior to the transverse process
35. They have transverse foramina and they are located more anteriorly on the vertebral arch, arising from the junction of the body and pedicle.
36. C-2
37. C-1
38. It is ringlike in structure, having no body or spinous process.
39. Lateral mass
40. Dens or odontoid process
41. Thoracic bodies are smaller, and more heart-shaped and bear facets for articulation with the ribs; lumbar bodies are larger and more cylindrical.
42. Superior articular processes
43. cervical = oblique
    thoracic = lateral
    lumbar = lateral
44. A smooth round or semicircular depression on the body of a thoracic vertebra for articulation with a rib
45. Thoracic
46. Pars interarticularis
47. nose = transverse process
    ear = superior articular process
    neck = pars interarticularis
    eye = pedicle
    front leg = inferior articular process

48. Base; apex
49. Five
50. Sacralization
51. Anterior and posterior sacral foramina
52. Alae
53. Sacral promontory
54. It is ear-shaped and is located on the posterolateral side of each ala.
55. Sacral hiatus
56. Lumbarization
57. Cartilage
58. Median sacral crest
59. 3–5
60. Cornua
61. More
62. Annulus fibrosis
63. Nucleus pulposus
64. Herniated nucleus pulposus
65. It is a cartilaginous (symphysis) joint classified as amphiarthrodial with slight movement.
66. The superior and inferior articular processes of adjacent vertebrae
67. A. AP open mouth
    B. lateral
    C. oblique
    D. oblique
68. Located between the vertebral bodies, they act as shock absorbers to cushion the vertebrae during movement.
69. Atlantoaxial joint (between C-1 and C-2)
70. Atlanto-occipital joint (between C-1 and the occipital bone)
71. Costovertebral
72. Costotransverse
73. Pivot (rotational movement)
74. A. 4
    B. 5
    C. 1
    D. 7
    E. 2
    F. 8
75. Removal of the immobilization devices may cause damage to the spinal cord if the neck is moved and an injury is present in this region of the vertebral column
76. 72 in.
77. The thinnest area should be placed under the anode. On an AP projection, the upper thoracic region (neck) is at the anode end, while the lower thoracic region (waist) is at the anode end on the lateral projection.
78. To place the spine parallel to the film plane and keep the intervertebral joints open
79. Lateral
80. To minimize the radiation dose to the radiosensitive breasts and gonads, particularly since this examination is frequently performed on young girls
81. To blur the overlying ribs and lung markings
82. Suspended expiration
83. 15–20° cephalad; C-4 (thyroid cartilage)
84. 45°
85. T-7 (3–4 in. below the jugular notch)
86. The vertebral bodies should appear boxlike; the pedicles of each vertebrae should be superimposed; the posterior ribs should be superimposed
87. 70°; 20°
88. Flexing the legs will lessen the lordotic curve of the lumbar spine, placing the spine closer to the table and positioning the intervertebral joint perpendicular to the film.

89. 45°
90. The level of the iliac crest
91. 2 in. medial to the elevated ASIS
92. Hyperflexion and hyperextension lateral projections
93. 35°; the ASIS
94. To reduce the amount of scatter reaching the film and to improve radiographic quality
95. 1½ in. posterior to the midaxillary line at a point midway between the level of the iliac crest and ASIS
96. A. sacrum = 15° cephalad
    B. coccyx = 10° caudal
97. Lateral
98. 2 in. superior to the symphysis pubis
99. A. LPO or RAO
    B. lateral
    C. lateral
    D. RPO or LAO
    E. RPO or LAO
    F. LPO or RAO
    G. AP
    H. lateral
    I. lateral
    J. AP
100.

Projection	CR Angle/Angle of Part	Centering Point	Film Size	Structures Seen
RPO cervical spine	CR = 15–20° cephalad part = 45°	C-4 (thyroid cartilage)	10 × 12 in. lw	Left intervertebral foramina and left pedicles; also the vertebral bodies of C2–T1 and intervertebral joints
LAO thoracic spine	CR = perpendicular part = 70° from PA or 20° from lateral	T-7 (tip of scapula)	14 × 17 in. lw	Left zygapophyseal joints; also the thoracic vertebral bodies and intervertebral joints
Lateral cervicothoracic region	CR = 3–5° caudal part = 90°	T-1	10 × 12 in. lw	Intervertebral joints (disk spaces) and vertebral bodies of C5–T4
LPO lumbar spine	CR = perpendicular part = 45° from AP or lateral	L-3 (1–1½ in. above iliac crest)	11 × 14 in. lw	Left zygapophyseal joints and "scotty dogs" (left pedicles, laminae, pars interarticulares, and articular processes)
Lateral coccyx	CR = perpendicular part = 90°	Palpate at base of spine	8 × 10 in. lw	Coccygeal segments and cornua (distal ⅓ of sacrum also included)

1. Either of two methods may be used to visualize this hypersthenic patient's lumbar spine. Radiolucent supports may be used to make the spine parallel with the table top, or the central ray may be angled 5–8° cephalic to compensate for the angle of the lumbar vertebrae when this hypersthenic patient lies in a lateral position. The angle of the L5–S1 spot could also be determined by drawing an imaginary line between the patient's iliac crests and directing the central ray parallel to that line. If the patient has spondylolisthesis, the defect would be visualized on the oblique radiographs as a radiolucent line in the pars interarticularis. The lateral radiograph would show if there is forward displacement of L-4 or L-5. If a herniated disk is the problem the nucleus pulposus will be herniated through the annulus pulposus posteriorly. This would possibly be visualized as a narrowed disk space on an AP radiograph. A herniated disk would also be more definitively visualized on a myelogram, a CT, or an MRI.

2. The sacrum and coccyx would have to be accomplished with the patient in the prone position. The usual angles would be reversed. A caudal angle would be used for the PA sacrum and a cephalic angle would be used for the PA coccyx. The central ray would be centered higher for the PA sacrum when done to replace the AP, and lower for the PA coccyx when done to replace the AP. If the patient was unable to lie on her side a cross-table lateral sacrum and coccyx could be done.

3. The AP thoracic spine would be done in the normal manner for the woman who fell from the balcony. The lateral and Swimmer's thoracic radiographs would have to be accomplished using a horizontal beam, however. The Swimmer's radiograph would require a cephalic angulation of 3–5° as it would be very difficult to sufficiently separate the patient's shoulders when she is lying in a supine position.

4. The technical factors for the extremely kyphotic woman should be decreased to compensate for her obvious osteoporosis. Both the AP and lateral thoracic spine could be easily accomplished if this woman is able to sit on a stool for the exam. The lateral could be accomplished with the patient positioned on her side, if she is unable to sit upright. It may be necessary to position the 14 × 17 in. film crosswise if her kyphosis is extreme. The AP thoracic spine could also be accomplished by leaving the patient in the lateral position and doing a left or right lateral decubitus using an AP projection.

5. Since the cervical spine of the patient involved in a motor vehicle accident has NOT been cleared, the rest of the series must be completed without moving the patient from the backboard or removing his cervical collar. The radiographs that would pose the greatest challenge would be the obliques. The oblique projections should be performed using a nongrid, table-top technique. The tube would be angled 45° cross-table and 15–20° cephalad. If the oblique cervical spine radiographs are for alignment rather than to see the intervertebral foramina, the tube would be angled 45° but no cephalic angulation would be necessary.

11 SKULL

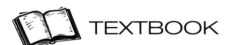 TEXTBOOK

Objectives:

Following the completion of this chapter, the student will be able to:

1. Given diagrams, radiographs, or dry bones, name and describe the bones of the skull.
2. Differentiate between the bones of the skull cap (calvarium) and the cranial floor.
3. Identify any surface markings and topographic landmarks found on the bones of the skull.
4. Using a lab partner or a drawing of the head, identify the localizing lines and planes used for radiographic positioning of the skull.
5. List any additional names for the structures of the skull.
6. Classify the articulations of the skull according to structure and function.
7. Differentiate between the three shape classifications of the skull, and discuss their implications on positioning of the petrous portions.
8. List and describe the basic projections of the skull, petrous portions, and mastoids, to include preferred type and size of image receptor, central ray location, and structures best visualized.
9. Practice positioning the basic projections of the skull, petrous portions, and mastoids on another student or phantom.
10. State the criteria used to determine positioning accuracy on radiographs of the skull, petrous portions, and mastoids.
11. Discuss the rationale for giving breathing instructions for radiographic examinations of the skull.
12. Evaluate radiographs of the skull in terms of positioning, centering, image quality, radiographic anatomy, and pathology.
13. Describe equipment considerations and exposure factors relative to radiography of the skull.
14. Describe positioning modifications that might be necessary depending upon a patient's body habitus.
15. Describe procedural adaptations necessary for radiography of the skull in a trauma situation.
16. Define terminology associated with the skull, to include anatomy, procedures, and pathology.

Chapter Outline

I. ANATOMY OF THE SKULL
- A. Calvarium
  1. frontal
  2. right and left parietal
  3. occipital

B. Floor
   1. ethmoid
   2. sphenoid
   3. right and left temporal
C. Ear
   1. external ear
   2. middle ear
   3. inner ear

II. ARTHROLOGY OF THE SKULL
   A. Sutures
      1. coronal
      2. sagittal
      3. lambdoidal
      4. squamosal
   B. Temporomandibular Joints
   C. Fontanels
      1. bregma
      2. lambda
      3. anterolateral (sphenoid)
      4. posterolateral (mastoid)

III. PROCEDURAL CONSIDERATIONS
   A. Patient Preparations
   B. Positioning Considerations
      1. routine/optional projections
      2. topographic landmarks
      3. positioning lines and planes
      4. skull morphology
   C. Trauma Considerations
   D. Alternate Projections
   E. Pediatric Radiography
   F. Breathing Instructions
   G. Exposure Factors
   H. Equipment Considerations

IV. RADIOGRAPHIC POSITIONING OF THE SKULL, PETROUS PORTIONS, MASTOIDS
   A. Skull: AP Axial, PA Axial, Lateral, Submentovertical, Verticosubmental,
      1. technical considerations
      2. shielding
      3. patient positioning
      4. part positioning
      5. central ray
      6. breathing instructions
      7. image evaluation
      8. critical anatomy
   B. Petrous Portions/Mastoids: Axiolateral, Axiolateral Oblique, Posterior Profile, Anterior Profile
      1. technical considerations
      2. shielding

      3. patient positioning

      4. part positioning

      5. central ray

      6. breathing instructions

      7. image evaluation

      8. critical anatomy

   V. SUMMARY

  VI. CRITICAL THINKING & APPLICATION QUESTIONS

 VII. FILM CRITIQUE

► SAMPLE 50-MINUTE LESSON

PREPARATION STEP   ESTIMATED TIME—10 MINUTES

A. Assemble teaching aids
   1. Overhead projector
   2. Overhead transparencies
      a. included in *Instructor's Resource Manual*
      b. trace drawings from *Applications Manual* on clear radiographic film
   3. Skeleton
   4. Radiographs
B. Introduce topic of anatomy of the skull. Lecture will include Chapter Objectives 1 to 4.
C. Opening discussion
   1. The bony anatomy of the skull is somewhat complicated and intricate. It is very important to have a thorough knowledge of each separate bone, any surface markings or parts that are named on that bone, plus where each bone is located within the skull.
   2. Even though CT has replaced the need for many skull radiographs, numerous positions/projections are still being performed on a regular basis in many imaging facilities.
   3. The first step to performing excellent skull and mastoid radiographs is to learn the anatomy very well. You must be able to describe and visualize the bones of the skull listed in the text.

PRESENTATION STEP   ESTIMATED TIME—40 MINUTES

TEACHING OUTLINE	TEACHING AIDS & METHODS
I. Skull	*Skull transparencies showing bones from different projections*
A. Composed of 22 Bones Plus 6 Auditory Ossicles	
1. 8 cranial bones	
2. 14 facial bones	
a. discussed further in next chapter	
B. Cranium	*Point out on skull*
1. calvarium	
a. frontal	
b. right parietal	
c. left parietal	
d. occipital	
2. floor	
a. sphenoid	
b. ethmoid	
c. right temporal	
d. left temporal	

II. Anatomy of the Bones of the Cranium
  A. Frontal
    1. anterior aspect of cranium
    2. divided into two main parts
      a. squamous portion/vertical portion
        (1) frontal tuberosity/eminence
        (2) superciliary ridge/arch
          (a) beneath the eyebrow
        (3) glabella
          (a) between eyebrows
        (4) frontal sinuses
          (a) behind glabella
        (5) supraorbital margin
          (a) upper rim of orbit
        (6) supraorbital foramen
          (a) medial to midpoint of supraorbital
             margin
      b. orbital portion/horizontal portion
        (1) orbital plates
          (a) from roof of orbits
        (2) ethmoid notch   *Reinforce how notch named for part*
          (a) opening between plates   *that fits into it*
          (b) cribriform of ethmoid fits into notch
        (3) articulates with lesser wings of sphenoid
  B. Parietal
    1. from lateral walls and roof of cranium
    2. parietal eminence
      a. tuberosity on lateral surface of skull
      b. widest dimension of skull between eminences
  C. Occipital
    1. forms posteroinferior wall and floor of cranium
    2. divided into four parts around foramen magnum
      a. squamous
        (1) curves upward from foramen magnum
        (2) forms posterior wall
        (3) articulates with parietal and temporal
           bones
        (4) external occipital protuberance
          (a) inion
          (b) bump on midline of back of head
      b. right and left lateral portions
        (1) lateral to foramen magnum
      c. basilar portion
        (1) located in front of foramen magnum
        (2) articulates with body of sphenoid
        (3) area where slopes forward to meet
           sphenoid called *clivus*
  D. Ethmoid
    1. located on midline of skull between orbits
    2. anterior to sphenoid
    3. divided into three parts   *Pass around ethmoid bones if*
      a. horizontal portion   *available*
        (1) cribriform plate
          (a) fits into ethmoid notch
          (b) contains olfactory nerves

        (2) crista galli

           (a) projects upward from cribriform plate

    b. vertical portion

        (1) perpendicular plate

           (a) forms superior portion of bony nasal septum

    c. lateral masses/labyrinths

        (1) suspended from underside of cribriform plate

        (2) contain 3–18 ethmoid air cells

        (3) superior and middle nasal concha or turbinate

           (a) project into nasal cavity from median wall of lateral masses

E. Sphenoid

    1. articulates with each of other seven cranial bones

    2. sits mid-cranium

    3. divided into three parts

    a. body

        (1) encloses sphenoid sinuses

        (2) sella turcica   *Draw sella on board*

           (a) saddle-shaped depression

           (b) houses pituitary gland

           (c) located ¾ in. anterior and ¾ in. superior to EAM on lateral skull

           (d) dorsum sellae

               (i) posterior border

           (e) posterior clinoid processes

               (i) project from lateral margin of dorsum sellae

           (f) tuberculum sellae

               (i) anterior border

        (3) optic groove

           (a) runs across body anterior to sella

    b. lesser wings

        (1) anterior clinoid processes

           (a) extend from posterior margin of lesser wings

    c. greater wings

        (1) posterior to lesser wings

    d. pterygoid processes   *Point out on skull*

        (1) project from underside of sphenoid at junction of body and greater wings

---

APPLICATION STEP   ESTIMATED TIME—2 HOURS

Study Assignment

A. Begin reading Chapter 11 in the text.

B. Begin Chapter 11 in the *Applications Manual.*

C. Name all the parts of the bones of the cranium on the skull of the skeleton.

D. Locate the anatomy discussed in class on the appropriate radiographs.

TESTING STEP

Questions on this material will be included in exam given at end of this chapter.

EXAM QUESTIONS ◄

Multiple Choice

1. You are viewing a submentovertical projection, which you just took as part of a skull series. Which of the following structures will be visualized on the radiograph?
   A. sphenoid sinus within the sphenoid bone
   B. crista galli of the ethmoid bone
   C. frontal bone with the orbital roofs superimposed
   D. styloid processes of the temporal bone

2. If you are doing a posterior profile (Stenvers) to see the IAC and your patient has a dolichocephalic skull in which the petrous pyramids form a 40° angle to the midsagittal plane, how many degrees should you oblique the skull?
   A. 40°
   B. 45°
   C. 50°
   D. 90°

3. The requisition calls for an AP axial (Towne) skull radiograph. Due to the patient's inability to tuck the chin, the IOML is perpendicular to the film rather than the OML. How would you compensate for this?
   A. angle the tube 23° caudad
   B. angle the tube 30° caudad
   C. angle the tube 37° caudad
   D. use no angle on the tube

4. The patient's nose and forehead are against the Bucky. The OML is perpendicular to the film and there is no angle on the CR. Where will the petrous pyramids be projected on your radiograph?
   A. below the maxillary sinuses
   B. in the lower third of the maxillary sinuses
   C. in the lower third of the orbits
   D. filling the orbits

5. The patient's nose and forehead are against the Bucky. The OML is perpendicular to the film and there is a 15° angle on the CR. Where will the petrous pyramids be projected on your radiograph?
   A. below the maxillary sinuses
   B. in the lower third of the maxillary sinuses
   C. in the lower third of the orbits
   D. filling the orbits

6. The line that must be perpendicular to the film when you are positioning for an AP skull is the
   A. OML
   B. IOML

C. MML

D. AML

7. Which of the following criteria must be met when performing a posterior profile radiograph (Stenvers) of the mastoids on a mesocephalic head?
   1. the head is positioned so it is resting on the nose, chin, and zygoma
   2. the median sagittal plane of the patient's head forms a 45° angle to the film
   3. there is a 12° cephalic angle on the CR

   A. 1 only

   B. 1 and 2 only

   C. 2 and 3 only

   D. 1, 2, and 3

8. You have positioned your patient's head in a true lateral. The CR is centered ¾ in. superior and ¾ in. anterior to the EAM. An extension cylinder is mounted on the tube. What anatomical part are you radiographing?

   A. down side TMJ

   B. sella turcica

   C. styloid process

   D. skull

9. The AP axial (Towne) skull is primarily done to visualize the

   A. parietal bones

   B. occipital bone

   C. frontal bone

   D. sphenoid bone

10. The patient's head is positioned so the medial sagittal plane forms a 15° angle to the plane of the film, and the CR is angled 15° caudal. What position/method is being described?

    A. posterior profile (Stenver)

    B. axiolateral (Schuller)

    C. transcranial (Schuller)

    D. modified lateral (Law)

11. Where is the sella turcica projected on an AP axial (Towne) radiograph when a 30° caudal angle is used and the patient's OML is perpendicular to the film?

    A. below the orbits

    B. within the orbits

    C. below the foramen magnum

    D. within the foramen magnum

12. The parts of the occipital bone that surround the foramen magnum are

    A. basilar portion, lateral portions, squamous portion

    B. greater wings, lesser wings, body

    C. squamous portion, orbital portion

    D. cribriform plate, lateral masses, perpendicular plate

13. Which part of which bone forms the superior portion of the bony nasal septum?

    A. horizontal portion of the frontal bone

    B. perpendicular portion of the ethmoid bone

C. the ethmoid notch in the frontal bone

D. the pterygoid process of the sphenoid bone

14. You are positioning a patient for a SMV radiograph and he is unable to bend back sufficiently so the IOML is parallel to the film. How would you compensate for this?

A. angle the CR until it is perpendicular to the IOML

B. angle the CR until it is parallel to the MML

C. angle the CR 30° caudad

D. angle the CR 37° caudad

15. A caliper measurement of the head taken between the parietal eminences would be most useful for which position/projection?

A. AP axial (Towne)

B. PA axial (Caldwell)

C. SMV

D. lateral

Answer Key

1. A	4. D	7. C	10. D	13. B
2. C	5. C	8. B	11. D	14. A
3. C	6. A	9. B	12. A	15. D

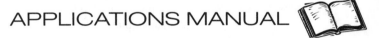

APPLICATIONS MANUAL

DRAWINGS ◄

It is very difficult to color each bone on the skull and mastoid drawings and so it is not required. Some students try to color each bone, some color the whole head, and some just label the parts. It is important, however, that the students label the angle of the CR and the degree of head rotation on the small head drawings that are included with each drawing.

ANSWER KEY FOR STUDY QUESTIONS ◄

1. The bony helmet that encloses and protects the brain, blood vessels, and nerves of the head; also called the brainbox

2. _____

Calvarium	Cranial Floor
Frontal	Sphenoid
Occipital	Ethmoid
Right parietal	Right temporal
Left parietal	Left temporal

_____

3. 8 cranial; 14 facial
4. Flat; irregular
5. Compact; cancellous
6. It is named for the middle layer of cancellous bone sandwiched between the inner and outer tables of the bones of the calvarium.
7. Squamous and orbital
8. Right and left parietal bones
9. Occipital
10. Ethmoid
11. Sphenoid
12. Temporal bone
13. Squamous (vertical)
14. Superciliary arches
15. These paired cavities are situated between the inner and outer tables of bone on the squamous portion of the frontal bone.
16. Orbital plates
17. Sphenoid
18. Ethmoidal notch
19. Parietal bones
20. Frontal tuberosities (eminences)
21. Parietal eminences (tuberosities)
22. Foramen magnum
23. External occipital protuberance (inion)
24. On the basilar portion of the occipital bone where it articulates with the sphenoid bone, specifically in the area between the foramen magnum and dorsum sellae
25. Superior and inferior nuchal lines
26. Occipito-atlantal joint
27. Horizontal; ethmoidal notch
28. They allow for the passage of the olfactory nerves, which are necessary for the sense of smell.
29. Crista galli
30. Lateral masses; labyrinths
31. Turbinates
32. Lateral masses (labyrinths)
33. They serve to warm, filter, and moisten inhaled air before it passes to the lungs.
34. Body
35. Tuberculum sellae; dorsum sellae
36. Lesser wings
37. Sella turcica
38. Greater wings
39. Pterygoid processes
40. Superior orbital fissure
41. Pituitary gland
42. Tympanic, mastoid, petrous, and squamous
43. Squamous
44. Styloid process
45. Mastoid process
46. Petrous; squamous
47. 47°
48. Auricle; pinna
49. Tympanic cavity
50. Tympanic membrane
51. Malleus, incus, stapes
52. The auditory tube (eustachian tube) opens into the tympanic cavity and serves to equalize the pressure between the external and middle portions of the ear, which is what occurred with the popping sensation.

53. A. external ear (external acoustic canal)
    B. internal ear through the round window
    C. internal ear through the oval window
    D. auditory tube (eustachian tube)
    E. aditus into the mastoid antrum
54. Bony labyrinth; membranous labyrinths
55. Cochlea
56. Semicircular canals
57. The fluid in the internal ear moves through the membranous labyrinth. Membranous coverings over the oval and round window separate the fluid from the air in the tympanic cavity.
58. A suture is a joint formed by the articulation of two or more cranial bones.
59. Coronal
60. Sagittal
61. Lambdoidal
62. Squamosal
63. Fibrous (synostoses); synarthrodial
64. Fontanel
65. A wormian bone is also known as a sutural bone; it is an oddly shaped bone that develops between the sutures of the cranium.
66. Bregma
67. Lambda
68. Anterior fontanel
69. Mastoid; asterion
70. Parietal, sphenoid, and temporal
71. Occipital
72. Ethmoid
73. Temporal
74. Temporal
75. Sphenoid
76. Ethmoid
77. Frontal
78. Temporal
79. Ethmoid
80. Occipital
81. Sphenoid
82. Sphenoid
83. Frontal
84. Occipital
85. Temporal
86. Dolichocephalic
87. Acanthion
88. Canthi
89. Nasion
90. Frontal
91. Glabella
92. Orbitomeatal line (OML)
93. Midsagittal (median) plane
94. 7°
95. 37° caudad
96. Vertex
97. The dorsum sellae should be demonstrated within the shadow of the foramen magnum.
98. 15° caudad
99. The distance between the outer margin of the orbits and lateral margin of the skull should be equal on both sides; the petrous portions of the temporal bones should be symmetrical.

100. Midway between the glabella and inion, which is approximately 2 in. above the EAM on a mesocephalic head
101. One orbital plate will be seen inferiorly to the other one instead of superimposed over each other
102. IOML—parallel
    midsagittal plane—parallel
    interpupillary line—perpendicular
103. Submentovertical projection (SMV)
104. Modified lateral (Law method)
105. Axiolateral oblique (Mayer method)
106. Lateral
107. Through the gonia
108. IOML
109. To help him/her hold still (prevent motion) and help maintain the position
110. 15°; 15° caudad
111. 45°; 45° caudad
112. Posterior profile (Stenver) projection for the petrous portions of the right temporal bone
113. Caudad
114.

Projection	CR Angle/ Angle of Part	Centering Point	Film Size	Structures Seen
PA skull	CR = 0° part = 0°	Nasion	10 × 12 in. lw	Vertical portion of frontal bone; petrous ridges filling entire orbits; also crista galli, frontal, and ethmoidal sinuses
Right axiolateral oblique (Mayer)	CR = 45° caudad part = 45°	Through the right EAM	8 × 10 in. cw	Mastoid air cells in right temporal bone; also EAM, bony labyrinth, and mastoid antrum
Left anterior profile (Arcelin)	CR = 10° caudad part = 45°	1 in. anterior to and ¾ in. superior to the left EAM (furthest from the film)	8 × 10 in. cw	Petrous ridge of right temporal bone parallel with the transverse axis of the film; internal acoustic canal, mastoid process, and mastoid air cells
Collimated lateral for sella turcica	CR = 0° part = 90°	¾ in. anterior and ¾ in. superior to EAM	8 × 10 in. cw	Horseshoe-shaped sella turcica, dorsum sellae, anterior and posterior clinoid processes
AP axial (Towne)	CR = 30° caudad to OML or 37° caudad to IOML part = 0°	Enters approx. 2½ in. above the superciliary arch and exits through foramen magnum	10 × 12 in. lw	Occipital bone, lambdoidal suture, and dorsum sellae within the foramen magnum

DISCUSSION OF ATYPICAL CASE STUDIES ◄

1. The skull projections that would most likely be taken on the 2-year-old child would be an AP, lateral, and AP axial. A tangential projection skimming over the wound could also be ordered if depression of the frontal bone were suspected. Since the injury is to the frontal bone, a PA skull radiograph could be attempted but would be very difficult on an upset 2-year-old. Most likely an AP, as well as the other projections, could be accomplished if the child's head were held securely by the mother (if there were no chance that she was pregnant.) Several wash cloths could be rolled together into two rolls that the mother could hold on each side of the child's head. The technologist should keep reassuring the child and direct the mother in a calm voice as the case progresses. If the mother is unable to take part in the exam or if the child is calmer without the mother in the room, a health care professional who is not a radiologic technologist should be asked to hold the child's head.

2. Performing a mastoid exam on an extremely kyphotic woman would be a very challenging exam. The exam could be accomplished most easily if the patient could sit upright on a stool for the exam. If this cannot be accomplished, her head could be built up on sponges until she was comfortable. This would increase the OID on most of the radiographs so the SID would have to be increased to decrease magnification of the skull. An AP projection would be used for the modified laterals so the direction of angulation of the CR would be reversed.

12 FACIAL BONES & PARANASAL SINUSES

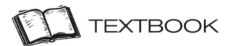 TEXTBOOK

Objectives:

Following the completion of this chapter, the student will be able to:

1. Given diagrams, radiographs, or dry bones, name and describe the bones of the face.
2. Discuss the location and structural makeup of the four groups of paranasal sinuses.
3. Identify the topographic landmarks associated with radiographic positioning of the facial bones.
4. Describe the bony construction of the orbits, to include a discussion of their shape and placement within the cranium, as well as their openings.
5. Classify the articulations of the facial bones according to structure and identify their type of movement, if applicable.
6. List and describe the basic projections of the facial bones, paranasal sinuses, and optic foramina, to include preferred type and size of image receptor, central ray location, and structures best visualized.
7. Practice positioning the basic projections of the facial bones, paranasal sinuses, and optic foramina on another student or phantom.
8. Explain the rationale for performing a radiographic examination of the paranasal sinuses in the upright position with a horizontal beam.
9. Describe procedural modifications that might be helpful when radiographing the facial bones in a trauma situation and when specific pathology is suspected.
10. Discuss the positioning modifications necessary to demonstrate either the ramus or the body of the mandible.
11. Discuss the rationale for radiographing the temporomandibular joints in both the open- and closed-mouth positions and differentiate between those positions on radiographs.
12. Describe equipment considerations and exposure factors relative to radiography of the facial bones, paranasal sinuses, and optic foramina.
13. State the criteria used to determine positioning accuracy on radiographs of the facial bones, paranasal sinuses, and optic foramina.
14. Evaluate radiographs of the facial bones, paranasal sinuses, and optic foramina in terms of positioning, centering, image quality, radiographic anatomy, and pathology.
15. Differentiate between "tri-pod" and "blow-out" fractures with regard to structures involved and radiographic projections on which each is best demonstrated.
16. Define terminology associated with the facial bones, paranasal sinuses, and optic foramina, to include anatomy, procedures, and pathology.

Chapter Outline

    B. Facial Bones: PA, Parietoacanthial, Lateral, Parieto-orbital Oblique
  1. technical considerations
  2. shielding
  3. patient positioning
  4. part positioning
  5. central ray
  6. breathing instructions
  7. image evaluation
  8. critical anatomy
    C. Nasal Bones: Lateral
    D. Zygomatic Arches: Submentovertical, Tangential, Superoinferior
    E. Mandible: PA Axial, Axiolateral Oblique, AP Axial
    F. Temporomandibular Joints: Axiolateral, Axiolateral Oblique
  VI. SUMMARY
  VII. CRITICAL THINKING & APPLICATION QUESTIONS
  VIII. FILM CRITIQUE

▶ SAMPLE 50-MINUTE LESSON

PREPARATION STEP   **ESTIMATED TIME—10 MINUTES**

  A. Assemble teaching aids
  1. Overhead projector
  2. Overhead transparencies
    a. included in *Instructor's Resource Manual*
    b. trace drawings from *Applications Manual* on clear radiographic film
  3. Skeleton
  4. Radiographs
  B. Introduce topic of anatomy of the paranasal sinuses and procedural considerations for facial bones and sinuses. Lecture will include Chapter Objectives 2, 8, and 9.
  C. Opening discussion
  1. The basic anatomy was discussed during the last class. We will be continuing with the objectives beginning with the anatomy of the paranasal sinuses. We will then continue with procedural considerations for positioning of facial bones and sinuses.
  2. You must learn many pieces of information extremely well to perform optimal radiographs of the facial bones and sinuses.

PRESENTATION STEP   **ESTIMATED TIME—40 MINUTES**

TEACHING OUTLINE	TEACHING AIDS & METHODS
I. Anatomy of the Paranasal Sinuses	*Transparency of sinuses*
A. Air-filled Cavities Located in	
1. frontal bone	
2. sphenoid bone	
3. ethmoid bone	
4. maxillary bone	
B. Mucous Lined Chambers That Are Continuous With the Nasal Cavity	

C. Begin to Form During Fetal Development
D. Grow to Become Cavities Formed Between Inner and Outer Tables
E. All Sinuses Communicate With and Drain Into the Nasal Cavity
F. Functions of Paranasal Sinuses
    1. lighten the skull
    2. warm and humidify air before passes to lungs
    3. intensify the resonance of the voice
G. Frontal Sinuses
    1. located behind glabella in squamous portion of frontal bone
    2. size and shape vary greatly so usually are not symmetrical
    3. may be divided into smaller compartments by multiple septa
    4. may be absent altogether
H. Ethmoid Sinuses
    1. located between the nasal cavity and each orbit
    2. located in lateral masses of ethmoid
    3. three groups of air cells in each lateral mass
        a. anterior
        b. middle
        c. posterior
    4. number of cells vary per area and individual
I. Sphenoid Sinuses
    1. located in body of sphenoid bone
    2. may or may not be paired depending on presence of thin bony septum
    3. located directly inferior to the sella
    4. because located so close to base of skull, blood or CSF may seep through a basal skull fracture into the sinus
        a. cross-table lateral will demonstrate fluid levels
J. Maxillary Sinuses
    1. located in the body of each maxilla
    2. also known as antra of Highmore
    3. symmetrical and pyramidal in shape
        a. appear boxlike in lateral, however
    4. roots of teeth are in close proximity to antral floors
    5. upper tooth infection can spread to maxillary sinus

II. Procedural Considerations
A. Clean Any Surface That Will Be in Contact With Patient's Face With Cleaning Solution
    1. do in patient's presence
B. Wash Your Hands Immediately Prior to Touching Patient's Head
C. Patient Preparation
    1. first check to be sure correct patient
    2. all metallic objects removed from head and neck area

Locate sinuses on appropriate sinus radiographs

Show radiographs with hairpins, braids, metallic objects

  3. hairpins, barrettes, and elastic bands removed
     from hair
  4. obtain pertinent patient history
D. Positioning Considerations
  1. most skull and facial bone radiographs can be
     performed with the patient either erect or
     recumbent
  2. sinus radiographs should be performed with the
     patient upright
     a. demonstrates air–fluid level

*Sinusitis radiograph showing
air–fluid levels*

  3. the affected side should be closest to the film
     when performing single laterals for sinuses and
     facial bones
  4. orbits
     a. may do modified parietoacanthial
        (1) OML 55° to plane of film

*Draw on board comparison of 37°
OML and 55° OML*

     b. include both orbits on parieto-orbital oblique
        radiographs
        (1) can evaluate orbital rim of orbit farthest
            away from film
  5. foreign body in the eye
     a. patient should close eyes and hold in fixed
        position during exposure
     b. CT and US frequently used
     c. MRI is *contraindicated*
  6. mandible
     a. patient condition often dictates alternate
        means of positioning
  7. TMJs
     a. done bilaterally with mouth open and closed

TMJ radiographs

     b. be sure films clearly marked
E. Trauma Considerations
  1. do not move head if associated skull or spine
     injury
  2. cross-table projections may be necessary if
     patient can't be moved or to look for air–fluid
     levels in sinuses due to trauma
  3. mandible
     a. image both sides
        (1) trauma may cause second fracture or TMJ
            dislocation
F. Alternate Projections
  1. panorex may be used for mandible
     a. must include mandible, TMJs, inferior
        portions of nasal fossa, and maxillary sinuses

*Transparency showing panorex
positioning and panorex
radiographs*

G. Breathing Instructions
  1. suspend respiration for all positions/projections
     of face and sinuses
H. Exposure Factors
  1. zygoma, nose, axiolateral oblique mandible
     a. no grid
     b. 50–60 kVp
  2. AEC not recommended for sinuses

I. Equipment Consideration
   1. zygoma, nose, axiolateral oblique mandible
      a. no grid
   2. other projections of face and sinuses
      a. grid

APPLICATION STEP   ESTIMATED TIME—2 HOURS

Study Assignment

A. Continue reading Chapter 12 in the text.
B. Continue Chapter 12 in the *Applications Manual.*
C. Be sure you can locate all the anatomy discussed on a skeleton and on a radiograph.

TESTING STEP

Questions on this material will be included in exam given at end of this chapter.

EXAM QUESTIONS ◄

Multiple Choice

1. You are evaluating the parietoacanthial (Waters) projection taken as part of a paranasal sinus series. Which of the following would cause you to repeat the projections?
   1. equidistance bilaterally between orbital cavities and lateral margins of skull
   2. distortion of frontal sinus
   3. petrous portions projected just below the maxillary sinuses
      A. 1 only
      B. 2 and 3 only
      C. 1, 2, and 3
      D. none of the above

2. For which two projections is the IOML used as a positioning line?
   A. parietoacanthial/PA axial
   B. lateral/submentovertical
   C. AP axial/PA
   D. modified parietoacanthial/modified PA axial

3. You have been asked to do a portable parietoacanthial (Waters) projection on a comatose patient
   who must remain in the supine position. How would you achieve the projection with the patient in
   this position?
   A. angle the tube cephalad until the central ray is approximately parallel to the patient's MML
   B. use a 50° caudal angle
   C. explain to the radiologist that you can perform this exam only when the patient is able to roll
      over
   D. position the patient for an AP axial (Towne) as an alternate projection

4. You are doing a facial series and the protocol book requests a PA axial (Caldwell) to visualize the orbital rims. What angle would you use on the CR?
   A. 0°
   B. 7°
   C. 15°
   D. 25°

5. You are critiquing a parieto-orbital oblique (Rhese) radiograph you have just completed to visualize the optic foramina. Since you have done only three parieto-oblique radiographs in your entire career, how can you be sure that you have positioned the patient correctly?
   A. the optic foramen visualizes in the lower outer quadrant of the orbit
   B. the optic foramen visualizes in the inner upper quadrant of the orbit
   C. the optic foramen is oval and exactly in the middle of the orbit
   D. the optic foramen is superimposed by the lateral orbital rim

6. For which two projections is the OML used as a positioning line?
   A. parietoacanthial/PA axial
   B. lateral/submentovertical
   C. parieto-orbital oblique/lateral nasal bones
   D. tangential zygomatic arches/AP axial

7. Which paranasal sinus radiograph is ordered when a general survey of the sinuses is desired?
   A. lateral
   B. modified parietoacanthial
   C. parietoacanthial
   D. SMV

8. Why is it essential to perform sinus radiographs with the patient erect?
   A. a 72 in. SID can be achieved
   B. it is more comfortable for the patient
   C. you would use a head unit that is designed to do upright radiographs
   D. to demonstrate air–fluid levels in the sinuses

9. Which sinuses fill with blood following a "blow-out" fracture?
   A. frontal
   B. maxillary
   C. ethmoid
   D. sphenoid

10. How would you describe the floor of the orbit on a patient who is correctly positioned for a modified parietoacanthial radiograph in which the OML forms a 55° angle with the plane of the film?
    A. approximately parallel to the film
    B. approximately perpendicular to the CR
    C. approximately parallel to the CR
    D. approximately lateral to the film

11. How is the head positioned for the axiolateral oblique radiograph of the body of the mandible?
    A. in a true lateral
    B. rotated 30° toward the film
    C. rotated 45° toward the film
    D. with the nose and forehead against the Bucky

12. You have just performed an SMV projection to visualize the patient's zygomas. How should the position of the patient's head be changed from the SMV for a tangential projection of the left zygomatic arch?
    A. rotated 15° toward the left side
    B. rotated 15° toward the right side
    C. keep the patient's head in the same position but center over the left arch
    D. the head should be tipped so the patient's OML is parallel to the film

13. How is the patient positioned for a parieto-orbital oblique radiograph?
    A. the nose, cheek, and forehead are against the table
    B. the OML in perpendicular to the table
    C. the acanthomeatal line is parallel with the transverse axis of the film, and the midsagittal plane forms a 53° angle with the plane of film
    D. the interpupillary is perpendicular to the table and the midsagittal plane is parallel to the table

14. Which radiographic exam is performed bilaterally with the patient's mouth open and closed?
    A. SMV for zygomatic arches
    B. parieto-orbital oblique for the right and left orbit
    C. PA mandible for the body of the mandible
    D. axiolateral for the TMJs

15. Which bony structure is located between the mandible and larynx in the anterior portion of the neck?
    A. thyroid cartilage
    B. hyoid bone
    C. antrum of Highmore
    D. ethmoid air cells

ANSWER KEY

1. D	4. D	7. C	10. C	13. C
2. B	5. A	8. D	11. B	14. D
3. A	6. A	9. B	12. A	15. B

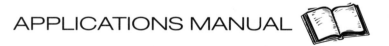

APPLICATIONS MANUAL

DRAWINGS ◀

The drawings in this chapter are also very difficult to color. The students should color each type of sinus a different color, however. As in the previous chapter it is important to reinforce that the students label the angle of the CR and the degree of head rotation on the small head drawings that are included with each drawing.

► ANSWER KEY FOR STUDY QUESTIONS

1. Right maxilla; left maxilla
   right zygomatic (malar); left zygomatic (malar)
   right nasal; left nasal
   right lacrimal; left lacrimal
   right palatine; left palatine
   right inferior nasal conchae; left inferior nasal conchae
   vomer; mandible
2. Maxillae
3. Palatine
4. Zygomatic (malar)
5. Lacrimal
6. Nasal
7. Inferior nasal conchae
8. Vomer
9. Mandible
10. Body
11. Infraorbital foramen
12. Lesser and greater wings of the sphenoid bone
13. Greater wing of the sphenoid and maxilla
14. Frontal
15. Alveolar
16. Palatal (palatine)
17. Zygomatic
18. Lacrimal
19. Palatine
20. Frontonasal; nasion
21. Malar
22. Tri-pod
23. Maxilla; ethmoid; frontal
24. Maxillary
25. Hard palate (maxillary and palatine bones)
26. Nasal septum
27. Symphysis menti
28. Rami
29. Mentum
30. Mental point
31. On the lateral aspects of the body of the mandible under the alveolar process
32. Gonion
33. Mandibular notch
34. Coronoid process
35. Condyle
36. Diarthrodial; hinge and gliding
37. Hyoid
38. Frontal, maxillary, and zygomatic
39. Frontal, maxilla, zygomatic, palatine, lacrimal, sphenoid, and ethmoid
40. Optic foramen
41. 30°; 37°
42. The maxilla in the floor of the orbit is fractured.
43. Modified parietoacanthial (Waters) projection
44. Gomphoses
45. Right and left temporomandibular joints (TMJ)
46. Forward

47. Frontal
48. Maxillary
49. Sphenoid
50. Ethmoid
51. Because the roots of the teeth are in close proximity to the antral floors
52. The side of interest should be radiographed. This can be determined from the patient's history.
53. To demonstrate air–fluid levels
54. Panorex (panoramic)
55. 15° caudad
56. The nasion
57. Parietoacanthial (Waters)
58. Frontal and ethmoidal air cells
59. ½–1 in. posterior to the outer canthus of the eye
60. Infraorbitomeatal line (IOML)
61. 25° caudad
62. The acanthion
63. The acanthion
64. 37°
65. 55°
66. Under the zygomatic bones
67. Midsagittal plane is parallel to the film plane, the interpupillary line is perpendicular to the film plane, and the IOML is parallel to the transverse axis of the film.
68. When the head is correctly positioned, the petrous ridges should be demonstrated just below the maxillary sinuses. When evaluating for rotation, the distance between the outer margin of the orbits and lateral margin of the skull should be equal and the petrous ridges should appear symmetrical.
69. 53°; right
70. Submentovertical (SMV)
71. 15°; toward; IOML
72. 20–25° cephalad
73. 30°; 15–25° cephalad
74. Approximately 1½ in. anterior and inferior to the TMJ of interest
75.

Projection	CR Angle/Angle of Part	Centering Point	Film Size	Structures Seen
PA sinuses	CR = 15° caudad part = 0°	Nasion	8 × 10 in. lw	Frontal and ethmoidal sinuses; petrous ridges seen in lower third of orbits; anterior ethmoidal sinuses seen above the petrous ridges
SMV for zygomatic arches	CR = perpendicular to IOML part = IOML parallel to film plane	At level of zygomatic arches (midway between gonia for bilateral arches)	8 × 10 in. cw	Zygomatic arches bilaterally free of superimposition

Continued

Projection	CR Angle/Angle of Part	Centering Point	Film Size	Structures Seen
Parietoacanthial (Waters) for facial bones	CR = 0° part = OML at 37° angle to film plane	Acanthion	8 × 10 in. lw	Orbital margins, zygomatic arches, coronoid processes of mandible, bony nasal septum; maxillary sinuses and gonia of mandible also demonstrated
Left lateral nasal bones	CR = 0° part = 90°	¾ in. inferior to nasion	8 × 10 in. cw	Superimposed nasal bones, frontonasal junction, anterior nasal spine of maxillae, and soft tissue structures of nose
Right axiolateral temporo-mandibular joint	CR = 25–30° part = 90°	TMJ nearest film	8 × 10 in. lw	Temporomandibular joint nearest film, including mandibular condyle and temporomandibular fossa of the temporal bone

► DISCUSSION OF ATYPICAL CASE STUDIES

1. A two- or three-view sinus series could be accomplished on the comatose patient even though she cannot be in an upright or prone position. The parietoacanthial projection would be changed to an acanthoparietal projection and the tube would be angled so that the CR is approximately parallel to the MML. The PA axial would be done as an AP axial with a cephalic angle on the tube. The amount of angulation would depend on the position of the patient's head. If the OML were perpendicular to the film, a 15° angle would be used. If the IOML were perpendicular to the film, a 22° angle would be used. The lateral should be done as a cross-table lateral to visualize any air–fluid levels in the sinuses that would indicate sinusitis. The areas of sinusitis would visualize as white on the radiograph. The maxillary sinuses would most likely be the ones affected.

2. The acanthoparietal would be done in the same manner as described above when radiographing the patient brought to the emergency department following a severe beating. It also would be very important to do a cross-table lateral to visualize any air–fluid levels in the sinuses, which would indicate bleeding. The SMV and tangential zygoma radiographs can easily be done with the patient on the table. The film is propped behind the patient's head and the tube is anterior to the patient's chest. If the films are not covered with a plastic bag, care must be taken to clean appropriately following the exam. The technologist should wear gloves and be aware of any areas that are touched during the exam.

INTRODUCTION TO CONTRAST STUDIES 13

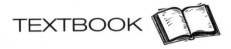

TEXTBOOK

Objectives:

Following the completion of this chapter, the student will be able to:

1. Discuss the term *contrast medium* to include its definition, its purpose, and its use in radiography.
2. Identify specific materials that are used as contrast agents, including the chemical, physical, and radiographic characteristics of each.
3. Differentiate between positive and negative contrast media.
4. Identify the routes of administration of contrast media for various radiographic examinations.
5. Compare and contrast the use of ionic and nonionic iodinated contrast media.
6. Identify contraindications for the administration of contrast media and possible complications resulting from its use.
7. Describe possible reactions to contrast media and categorize them according to severity.
8. Describe how contrast examinations differ from noncontrast examinations.
9. Describe the radiographer's responsibilities with regard to contrast examinations.
10. Describe the room preparation required for contrast examinations.
11. Identify appropriate methods of radiation protection for fluoroscopic procedures.
12. Discuss recommended sequencing of various diagnostic examinations and provide a rationale for this sequencing.

Chapter Outline

    I. BASIC PRINCIPLES OF CONTRAST MEDIA
       A. Contrast Media
          1. enhance the contrast of soft tissue structures by altering their density
   II. TYPES OF CONTRAST MEDIA
       A. Negative Contrast Media
          a. room air
          b. oxygen
          c. carbon dioxide
          d. nitrous oxide
       B. Positive Contrast Media
          1. barium sulfate
             a. properties
             b. contraindications

    2. iodinated compounds

       a. properties

       b. contraindications

III. ROUTE OF ADMINISTRATION

    A. Orally/Rectally

    B. Intravascularly

    C. Directly

IV. REACTIONS TO CONTRAST MEDIA

    A. Anaphylactoid

    B. Vasovagal

V. RELATED TERMINOLOGY

VI. PROCEDURAL CONSIDERATIONS

    A. Radiographer's Responsibilities

       1. patient preparation

       2. room preparation

       3. fluoroscopy

       4. radiation protection

VII. SEQUENCING OF EXAMINATIONS

VIII. SUMMARY

IX. CRITICAL THINKING & APPLICATION QUESTIONS

X. FILM CRITIQUE

► SAMPLE 50-MINUTE LESSON

PREPARATION STEP   ESTIMATED TIME—10 MINUTES

    A. Assemble teaching aids

       1. Overhead projector

       2. Overhead transparencies

         a. included in *Instructor's Resource Manual*

       3. Radiographic contrast studies

       4. Bottles of various iodine contrast media

       5. Different types of barium products

       6. Effervescent agents

    B. Introduce topic of contrast media and contrast studies. Lecture will include chapter objectives 1 to 6.

    C. Opening discussion

       1. Contrast media help visualize soft tissue structures in the body that are not readily visible on a radiograph.

       2. Contrast media are used to demonstrate structures of the urinary, digestive, and biliary system as well as the spinal canal, female reproductive system, and vasculature.

       3. Contrast media may be introduced into the body in various ways—by mouth, by rectum, by injecting into the veins, by retrograde filling of the bladder through an urinary catheter.

       4. It is important to *not* become complacent when injecting iodine contrast medium as it is possible for the patient to have a life-threatening reaction to it.

PRESENTATION STEP	ESTIMATED TIME—40 MINUTES

TEACHING OUTLINE	TEACHING AIDS & METHODS

I. Basic Principles of Contrast Media
  A. Contrast Media Helps Visualize Structures That Have Similar Densities Within the Body
II. Types of Contrast Media
  A. Negative Contrast Agent
    1. radiolucent/dark on radiograph
    2. has a low atomic number
    3. allows x-rays to pass through easily
    4. examples
       a. room air is most common   *Syringe with room air*
       b. O_2, CO_2, nitrous oxide
    5. may be used alone in study
       a. air arthrogram
    6. may be combined with positive contrast agent   *Radiograph of double-contrast study*
       to produce double-contrast effect
       a. barium enema exam with air
  B. Positive Contrast Agent   *Example of BE equipment used for air contrast*
    1. radiopaque/light on radiograph
    2. high atomic number
    3. absorbs 3 times more x-rays than bone
    4. examples
       a. iodine   *Example of iodine*
       b. barium sulfate   *Example of barium*
  C. Barium Sulfate
    1. insoluble in water
    2. inert compound
    3. used in alimentary canal
       a. administered orally
       b. administered rectally
    4. heavy metal with atomic number of 56
    5. contraindications
       a. cannot be used intravascularly
       b. cannot be used intrathecally
       c. cannot be used if suspected perforation in the alimentary canal or recent or impending abdominal surgery
  D. Iodinated Compounds
    1. atomic number of 53
    2. concentration of iodine affects viscosity
    3. types of iodinated compounds
       a. oil-based iodinated contrast media
          (1) fatty-acid base
          (2) insoluble in water
          (3) slowly absorbed
          (4) used in studies of lymphatic system
          (5) replaced by nonionic water-soluble contrast media in many exams today
       b. water-soluble iodinated contrast media
          (1) used in studies of the urinary, biliary, and cardiovascular systems

    (2) used in studies of digestive system when barium contraindicated

    (3) administered orally, rectally, intravascularly, or directly

    (4) *ionic* contrast agent

     (a) organic iodine compound

     (b) has triiodinated benzoic acid as its base

     (c) separates in water into two electrically charged particles

      (i) cation—positive

      (ii) anion—negative

    (5) *nonionic* contrast agent

     (a) more soluble in water

     (b) does *not* separate into charged particles

     (c) lower osmolality than ionic

    (6) osmolality

     (a) number of particles in the solution per kilogram of water

     (b) ionic: 1,000–24,000 osmoles/kg

      (i) can cross blood–brain barrier

       (a) factor in occurrence of adverse reactions

     (c) nonionic: 750 osmoles/kg

      (i) much lower level of neurotoxicity

      (ii) 6 times more costly

      (iii) approx. ⅓ fewer adverse reactions than with ionic

  4. contraindications

   a. allergic history to iodine

    (1) may premedicate with steroids or antihistamines

   b. anuria

   c. high creatinine level renal disease and other conditions that compromise renal function

    (1) diabetes mellitus

    (2) multiple myeloma

    (3) sickle-cell anemia

    (4) pheochromocytoma

   d. congestive failure

   e. severe dehydration

III. Routes of Administration

 A. The *Five Rights*

  1. the *right patient* should receive

  2. the *right medication*

  3. in the *right amount*

  4. via the *right route*

  5. at the *right time*

 B. Depends on Anatomy of Interest, Type of Exam, and Particular Contrast Media

 C. Oral

  1. esophagus, stomach, small intestine, and gallbladder exams   *Radiographic example of each*

   D. Rectal
      1. large intestine exams
   E. Intravenous
      1. excretory urography, IV cholangiography, CT,
         MRI exams
   F. Direct
      1. cystography
      2. myelography, arthrography
      3. hysterosalpingography, sialography
      4. percutaneous transhepatic cholangiography

APPLICATION STEP   ESTIMATED TIME—1 HOUR

Study Assignment

A. Read Chapter 13 in the text.
B. Complete Chapter 13 in the *Applications Manual.*

TESTING STEP

Questions on this material will be included in exam given at end of this chapter.

EXAM QUESTIONS ◄

Multiple Choice

1. Which type of contrast agent causes a radiolucent image on the radiograph due to its low atomic
   number?
   A. negative
   B. positive

2. The most common type of a negative contrast agent is
   A. barium sulfate
   B. iodinated compounds
   C. room air
   D. O_2

3. What is the purpose of administering effervescent agents during a study of the upper gastrointestinal system?
   A. so the stomach will absorb 3 times more x-rays and look light on the radiograph
   B. it forms CO_2 when mixed with water, which adds a negative contrast agent
   C. to relieve the patient's heartburn caused by the barium sulfate
   D. to cause the barium sulfate to go through the system faster

4. Which type of reaction occurs in response to anxiety or fear, and causes pallor, dizziness, diaphoresis, nausea, and possibly bradycardia?
   A. anaphylactoid reaction
   B. extravasation reaction
   C. nonionic contrast reaction
   D. vasovagal reaction

5. Which type of reaction closely resembles a true allergic reaction in which the patient demonstrates hypersensitivity when a foreign substance is injected?
   A. anaphylactoid reaction
   B. vasovagal reaction
   C. negative contrast reaction
   D. extravasation reaction

Please number the following exams from 1 to 5 in the order in which they should occur so that each exam does not compromise the success of the other diagnostic tests (i.e., exam 1 should be performed before exam 2, etc.).

6. _____ PA and lateral CXR

7. _____ Upper gastrointestinal study

8. _____ Barium enema

9. _____ Excretory urogram (IVP)

10. _____ Oral cholecystogram

11. What type of iodinated contrast medium should be used if the patient has a history of allergies, or seems very anxious about the exam?
    A. oil-based iodine
    B. ionic iodine
    C. nonionic iodine
    D. fat-soluble iodine

12. Which adverse reactions to iodinated contrast media are considered nuisance reactions and seldom require medical intervention?
    1. hot flash or flush
    2. metallic taste in mouth
    3. nausea/vomiting
       A. 1 and 2 only
       B. 1 and 3 only
       C. 2 and 3 only
       D. 1, 2, and 3

13. The term that refers to the concentration or number of particles in the solution per kilogram of water is
    A. diaphoresis
    B. osmolality
    C. toxicity
    D. miscibility

14. What area on the anterior side of the arm is commonly used for intravenous injection of contrast media?
    A. popliteal region
    B. olecranon region
    C. antecubital region
    D. coracoid region

15. An example of a severe contrast medium reaction that calls for immediate medical intervention is
    A. coughing and sneezing
    B. respiratory arrest
    C. itching
    D. hot flash or flush

ANSWER KEY

1. A	4. D	7. 5	10. 3	13. B
2. C	5. A	8. 4	11. C	14. C
3. B	6. 1	9. 2	12. D	15. B

APPLICATIONS MANUAL

ANSWER KEY FOR STUDY QUESTIONS ◄

1. A pharmaceutical agent that is administered to a patient for a radiographic examination to enhance the contrast of a particular structure
2. Because structures and organs of these systems have similarly low tissue densities and are not easily differentiated from surrounding structures without the aid of a contrast medium
3. Radiolucent
4. Room air; also, carbon dioxide, nitrous oxide, oxygen
5. Room air is used to inflate the lungs on inhalation. The lungs appear dark, while the adjacent ribs and vertebrae appear light.
6. More
7. Barium sulfate ($BaSO_4$)
8. Higher; lighter
9. $BaSO_4$ is not water-soluble and cannot be absorbed by the body.
10. Iodine-containing compounds
11. Low; high
12. Insoluble
13. Lymphatic system
14. It is very slowly absorbed by the body.
15. It mixes with blood and body fluids.
16. 3
17. Kidneys (urinary system); 24
18. Osmolality
19. Anion; cation
20. The nonionic contrast medium is more water-soluble and does not dissociate into charged particles; it also has a lower osmolality than ionic contrast agents and a lower level of neurotoxicity.
21. Iodine
22. There is less interruption of homeostasis and therefore fewer reactions when an injected contrast agent more closely resembles the osmolality of blood plasma. The osmolality of nonionic contrast medium is more similar to blood plasma than that of ionic contrast medium.
23. Any of the following: history of previous adverse reactions, history of cardiac impairment, history of allergies and/or asthma, increased patient anxiety, sickle-cell disease, generalized debilitation, or the patient requests it
24. 3
25. The radiologist
26. The anatomy of interest, the type of examination, and the particular type of contrast medium
27. Oral and rectal administration
28. Intravascular
29. Any of the following: cystogram, sialogram, arthrogram, percutaneous transhepatic cholangiography, or hysterosalpingogram
30. Hemodynamic changes occur when the contrast medium is injected, causing a disruption of homeostasis.
31. Anaphylactoid
32. Extravasation

33. Vasovagal
34. Mild (minor), moderate, and severe
35. Severe
36. Mild (minor)
37. Urticaria
38. What will happen during the exam; who will be involved in the procedure; what contrast medium will be used and how it will be administered; any possible side effects to the contrast medium; and the length of the examination
39. Emergency box/crash cart; disposable gloves; emesis basin; towels, sheets, blankets
40. I could pick up germs from being in contact with dirty equipment (nosocomial illness). I might question if the radiographer is organized and competent since the room appears unkempt.
41. Place the foot board on the table; move the Bucky tray to the foot of the table; turn the table upright (depending upon the patient's condition); place the foot switch in an accessible location; adjust the lead drape on the fluoro unit; load a cassette into the spot film device or prepare any other image recording device.
42. 5
43. Wear a lead apron with a thyroid collar; wear lead gloves; place a lead shield on the end of table under the infant's head
44. A. ultrasound examination of the gallbladder
    B. oral cholecystogram
    C. UGI
45. Yes; the excretory urogram would be performed first because the iodinated contrast medium is easily excreted from the kidneys, whereas residue from the barium sulfate might create unwanted artifacts and obscure anatomy.
46. True
47. False; these are both positive contrast media. In a double-contrast study, both negative and positive contrast agents are administered.
48. False; although the radiographer may administer the contrast medium in an examination, he/she is doing so upon the physician's orders.
49. True
50. True

WORD SEARCH

```
P C I M A N Y D O M E H C K B
H R A S N I O D I N A T E D R
A S I S A T S O E M O H O I Z
R M H Y P E R V O L E M I A N
M N I I H N L E T C T G X P L
A E Z M Y K A P N O O V A H T
C H N R L J G F E M X M I O D
E X T R A V A S A T I O N R K
U C C J C Y V W Z L C C F E T
T L F X T B O L U S I V U S N
I L W F O X S R B N T Y S I Q
C C K V I J A I O B Y Y I S Q
A B B C D D V I V H S J O Q B
L E E R A E J X O O A V N R R
```

WORD LIST

1. ANAPHYLACTOID
2. VASOVAGAL
3. PHARMACEUTICAL
4. HYPERVOLEMIA
5. HOMEOSTASIS
6. EXTRAVASATION
7. DIAPHORESIS
8. BOLUS
9. TOXICITY
10. HEMODYNAMIC
11. IONIC
12. INFUSION

14 URINARY SYSTEM

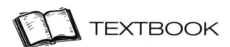 TEXTBOOK

Objectives:

Following the completion of this chapter, the student will be able to:

1. Given diagrams or radiographs, name and describe the anatomy of the urinary system, to include the kidneys, ureters, urinary bladder, and urethra.
2. Identify the functions of each of the structures in the urinary system.
3. Describe the vascular structures associated with each kidney.
4. Discuss the microscopic structure of the kidney and its role producing urine.
5. Discuss the relationship of the adrenal and prostate glands to the urinary system with regard to location.
6. Identify the key function of the urinary system and explain why it is vital for a person's health and well-being.
7. Discuss the physiologic process of producing urine.
8. Define *nephrolith* and *renal calculus* and identify the areas along the urinary tract where they are most likely to get "stuck."
9. Describe patient preparation and care relative to radiographic examination of the urinary tract.
10. Discuss the use of contrast media in radiographic examinations of the urinary tract, to include type and route of administration.
11. List and describe the basic projections for examinations of the urinary tract, to include preferred type and size of image receptor, central ray location, and structures best demonstrated.
12. Differentiate between functional and nonfunctional radiographic examinations of the urinary tract.
13. Practice positioning and basic projections of the urinary tract on another student or phantom.
14. Describe the breathing instructions for radiographic examinations of the urinary tract.
15. State the criteria used to determine positioning accuracy on radiographs of the urinary tract.
16. Evaluate radiographs of the urinary tract in terms of positioning, centering, image quality, radiographic anatomy, and pathology.
17. Describe equipment considerations and exposure factors relative to radiography of the urinary tract.
18. Identify alternative methods for evaluating the urinary system.
19. Describe how radiography of the urinary system should be modified for the pediatric patient.
20. Define terminology associated with the urinary tract, to include anatomy, procedures, and pathology.

Chapter Outline

I. ANATOMY OF URINARY SYSTEM
   A. Kidneys
      1. gross anatomy
      2. physiology
      3. blood supply
   B. Ureters
   C. Urinary Bladder
   D. Urethra

II. RELATED TERMINOLOGY

III. PROCEDURAL CONSIDERATIONS
   A. Patient Preparation
      1. exam preparation
   B. Room Preparation
   C. Positioning Considerations
   D. Alternate Projections/Procedures
   E. Pediatric Urography
   F. Breathing Instructions
   G. Exposure Factors
   H. Equipment Considerations

IV. RADIOGRAPHIC POSITIONING
   A. Excretory Urogram: AP Abdomen, AP Kidneys, AP Oblique Urinary Tract
      1. technical considerations
      2. shielding
      3. patient positioning
      4. part positioning
      5. central ray
      6. breathing instructions
      7. image evaluation
      8. critical anatomy
   B. Cystogram: AP, AP Oblique Urinary Bladder
      1. technical considerations
      2. shielding
      3. patient positioning
      4. part positioning
      5. central ray
      6. breathing instructions
      7. image evaluation
      8. critical anatomy

V. SUMMARY

VI. CRITICAL THINKING & APPLICATION QUESTIONS

VII. FILM CRITIQUE

► SAMPLE 50-MINUTE LESSON

PREPARATION STEP	ESTIMATED TIME—10 MINUTES

A. Assemble teaching aids
1. Overhead projector
2. Overhead transparencies
   a. included in *Instructor's Resource Manual*
3. Urinary system exam equipment
4. Anatomic model
5. Radiographs

B. Introduce topic of procedural considerations for radiographic examinations of the urinary system. Lecture will include Chapter Objectives 9 and 10.

C. Opening discussion
1. The anatomy and positioning of urinary system is very direct as there are no complicated positions to learn. The most important consideration when visualizing the urinary system is the patient's condition. There is no room for complacency when performing exams using iodinated contrast media.
2. Urography is a general term used to describe radiography of the urinary system. This visualization is accomplished by injecting iodinated contrast media into a vein or into a catheter that has been introduced into the structure to be studied.
3. Radiographic examination of the urinary system is performed to evaluate function, location of structures, and pathologic conditions.

PRESENTATION STEP	ESTIMATED TIME—40 MINUTES

TEACHING OUTLINE	TEACHING AIDS & METHODS
I. Procedural Considerations	*Transparency of anatomy*
A. Excretory Urogram (ExU)/Intravenous Pyelogram (IVP)/Intravenous Urogram (IVU)	*IVP radiographs*
1. series of radiographs taken at timed intervals after injection of contrast	
2. evaluates function, size, shape, and position of urinary structures	
B. Nephrogram	
1. nephron or "blush" phase when contrast seen in kidney parenchyma	*Radiographs of nephron stage*
2. radiographs should be obtained within one minute of the injection to visualize	
3. hypertensive IVP	
a. rapid injection and filming	
b. right and left kidney function compared	
c. if renal function different, may be result of renal artery stenosis, which can contribute to renal hypertension	
C. Infusion Urogram	
1. may be ordered if patient has impaired renal function indicated by lab values for serum creatinine and BUN	
a. normal lab values	
(1) serum creatinine	
(a) female 0.6–1.5 mg/100 mL	
(b) male 0.7–1.6 mg/100 mL	
(2) BUN	
(a) 6–17 g/day	

D. Retrograde Pyelogram
   1. visualized internal structures of kidneys and ureters
   2. ureteral catheter placed at the lower level of renal pelvis with assist of cystoscope
   3. allows identification and removal of calculi
   4. nonfunctional exam as does not demonstrate renal parenchyma
E. Cystogram
   1. exam of urinary bladder
   2. demonstrates shape and position
   3. demonstrates vesicoureteral reflux
F. Voiding Cystourethrogram (VCUG)
   1. cystogram followed by obtaining radiograph while patient voiding
   2. demonstrates lower urinary tract obstruction
   3. demonstrates vesicoureteral reflux
G. Patient Preparation
   1. preliminary preparation
      a. low-residue diet for 1–2 days before exam
      b. light meal night before exam
      c. non-gas producing cathartic evening before exam
      d. NPO (except water) after midnight day of exam
      e. intestines should be cleaned
      f. patient should NOT be dehydrated
   2. exam preparation
      a. identify patient
      b. have patient put on gown
      c. obtain pertinent history   *Transparency of history sheet*
      d. explain procedure to patient
      e. patient should void before exam
      f. if patient has urinary catheter, clamp before injecting contrast
   3. room preparation
      a. usual room preparation
      b. prepare contrast medium
      c. set out equipment for delivery of contrast   *Example of items necessary for exam*
         medium
      d. set out other supplies
         (1) compression device
         (2) emesis basin
         (3) emergency box for reactions
H. Positioning Considerations
   1. ExU/IVP   *IVP radiographs*
      a. scout film prior to contrast
         (1) proper exposure factors
         (2) proper positioning
         (3) presence of calculi
      b. positions of patient
         (1) supine
         (2) oblique
            (a) 30° LPO and RPO
         (3) prone
         (4) upright

           (5) Trendelenburg

    c. delayed films may be necessary if filling of ureter is slow

    d. compression device may be used

        (1) keeps contrast in kidneys

        (2) contraindications

            (a) ureteral stones

            (b) abdominal mass

            (c) abdominal aortic aneurysm

            (d) abdominal pain or trauma

            (e) recent abdominal surgery

            (f) pelvic kidney

            (g) colostomy

            (h) suprapubic catheter

2. Retrograde pyelogram

    a. scout before or after catheter(s) inserted

    b. radiograph of renal pelvis

    c. radiograph as catheter withdrawn

    d. positions of patient

        (1) supine

        (2) shallow oblique

    e. no contrast media injected when exam is for stone retrieval

3. Cystogram

    a. imaging may be done with fluoroscopic spots and/or overhead films

    b. positions of patient

        (1) AP with 15° caudal angle

        (2) 40–60° LPO and RPO to see UVJ

        (3) post-void AP

4. Voiding cystourethrogram

    a. voiding under fluoroscopy

    b. positions of patient

        (1) female supine or slight oblique

        (2) male 30° PRO

APPLICATION STEP   ESTIMATED TIME—2 HOURS

Study Assignment

A. Continue reading Chapter 14 in the text.

B. Continue Chapter 14 in the *Applications Manual.*

C. Be sure you can locate all the anatomy discussed on an anatomic model and on a radiograph.

D. Make sure you can differentiate the various exams of this system on the radiographs.

TESTING STEP

Questions on this material will be included in exam given at end of this chapter.

EXAM QUESTIONS ◄

Multiple Choice

1. Which radiographic exam of the urinary system evaluates function, structure, and pathologic conditions of the kidneys?
   A. retrograde pyelogram
   B. cystogram
   C. voiding cystourethrogram
   D. excretory urogram

2. What phase of kidney function is visible shortly after a venous injection of iodinated contrast medium?
   A. pyelogram
   B. nephrogram
   C. ureterogram
   D. cystogram

3. Which of the following contraindicates an excretory urogram?
   1. renal calculi
   2. recent abdominal surgery
   3. abnormally high levels of serum creatinine and blood urea nitrogen
   A. 1 only
   B. 3 only
   C. 1 and 2 only
   D. 1, 2, and 3

4. Which of the following contraindicates the use of compression during an excretory urogram?
   1. renal calculi
   2. an abdominal mass
   3. the presence of a pelvic kidney
   A. 1 only
   B. 3 only
   C. 1 and 2 only
   D. 1, 2, and 3

5. What is the purpose of angling the tube caudad for radiography of the urinary bladder?
   A. to prevent superimposition of the bladder neck by the symphysis pubis
   B. to help visualize the vesicoureteral region
   C. to help visualize the superior aspect of the urinary bladder
   D. to prevent superimposition of the symphysis pubis by the patient's thighs

6. What is the purpose of obtaining a scout film during an excretory urogram?
   1. to evaluate proper exposure factors
   2. to determine if radiopaque calculi are present
   3. to determine if the kidneys have picked up the contrast
   A. 2 only
   B. 3 only
   C. 1 and 2 only
   D. 1, 2, and 3

7. What is the main reason for using ureteral compression during an excretory urogram?
   A. to prevent the patient from breathing
   B. to immobilize the patient
   C. to promote filling of the renal calyces and pelves
   D. to aid in excretion

8. What is the purpose of rotating the patient 30° when obtaining oblique kidney radiographs?
   A. to place the elevated kidney parallel to the film
   B. to place the down-side kidney parallel to the film
   C. to radiograph the elevated kidney at a 30° angle to the film
   D. to radiograph the down-side kidney at a 30° angle to the film

9. Which radiograph taken during an excretory urogram would demonstrate the mobility of the kidneys?
   A. right lateral recumbent
   B. left lateral recumbent
   C. prone
   D. upright

10. Which exam should be performed first if a VCUG and excretory urogram are scheduled on the same day?
    A. the order of these two exams is not important, either can be done first
    B. the VCUG should be performed before the excretory urogram
    C. the excretory urogram should be performed before the VCUG
    D. these exams can *not* be performed on the same day under any circumstances

11. Why are all radiographs of the urinary system obtained during suspended expiration?
    1. to elevate the diaphragm to its highest position
    2. to prevent compression of abdominal contents
    3. to reduce tissue thickness of the patient
       A. 1 only
       B. 1 and 2 only
       C. 2 and 3 only
       D. 1, 2, and 3

12. To enhance subject contrast, what optimal kVp range should be used when performing an excretory urogram on an adult?
    A. 60–75 kVp
    B. 70–75 kVp
    C. 80–85 kVp
    D. 90–95 kVp

13. Where is the centering point for an AP collimated renal area radiograph?
    A. on the iliac crest
    B. on the xiphoid process
    C. halfway between the xiphoid process and iliac crest
    D. halfway between the symphysis pubis and iliac crest

14. Where is the centering point for an AP radiograph of the urinary bladder?
    A. 2 in. superior to the symphysis pubis on the midline of the body
    B. 1 in. inferior to the symphysis pubis on the midline of the body

C. at the level of the iliac crest on the midline of the body

D. at the level of the symphysis pubis on the midline of the body

15. Where is a renal calculi most likely to become lodged in the urinary system?

    A. in the minor calyx

    B. in renal pelvis

    C. at the ureterovesical junction

    D. in the urinary bladder

ANSWER KEY

1. D	4. D	7. C	10. B	13. C
2. B	5. A	8. A	11. D	14. A
3. B	6. C	9. D	12. B	15. C

APPLICATIONS MANUAL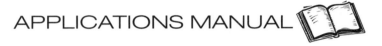

ANSWER KEY FOR STUDY QUESTIONS ◄

1. 2 kidneys, 2 ureters, 1 urinary bladder, and 1 urethra
2. Kidneys
3. The urinary system regulates the volume, pH, and concentration of organic waste products in the blood, and also helps control blood pressure.
4. The kidneys are located laterally to the vertebral column in the region between T-12 and L-3.
5. Psoas major; 20°
6. Posteriorly
7. 30°
8. Right; the presence of the liver causes it to be lower than the left kidney.
9. Renal hilum
10. The kidney is arbitrarily divided into upper and lower regions at the area of the hilum. Each region is referred to as a pole.
11. Adipose capsule
12. This refers collectively to the cortex and medulla, which comprise the functional tissue of the kidney.
13. Cortex
14. This is the innermost covering of the kidney and is adjacent to the kidney tissue.
15. The presence of the adipose capsule (perirenal fat)
16. Papillae
17. 8–18; medulla
18. Major calyces and minor calyces
19. Renal pyramids
20. Ureter
21. Urinary bladder
22. Nephron
23. Glomerulus
24. Filtration, reabsorption, and secretion
25. Glomerular (Bowman's) capsule
26. This term refers collectively to the glomerulus and glomerular capsule.
27. The capillaries forming the glomerulus have thin, semipermeable walls, which allow these substances to filter through them.

28. 95% water and 5% solid waste substances
29. 1–2 liters
30. Renal tubule
31. Renal artery
32. Renal calculus and nephrolith
33. To convey urine from the kidneys to the urinary bladder
34. Posterolateral
35. Peristalsis
36. Ureteropelvic junction, brim of the pelvis, and ureterovesical junction
37. Shock wave lithotripsy
38. Symphysis pubis; vagina
39. The kidneys and ureters are behind the peritoneum (retroperitoneal) and the urinary bladder is inferior to the peritoneum (infraperitoneal).
40. Rugae
41. Trigone
42. Micturition
43. Incontinence
44. Urethra
45. The entrances of each ureter and the urethra
46. Reproductive
47. Cystitis
48. Urography
49. External urethral orifice
50. The function of the urinary system can be examined as contrast medium is injected intravenously, filtered from the bloodstream, and excreted by the kidneys.
51. Nephrograms
52. A hypertensive study is performed on a patient with high blood pressure to determine if the kidneys are responsible for the hypertension. Differences in renal function between the kidneys may be attributed to renal artery stenosis.
53. Creatinine is a waste product normally excreted by the kidneys. If the creatinine level in the blood is high, renal function is impaired. In this case, the injection of contrast media may damage kidney tissue.
54. Retrograde pyelogram
55. Vesicoureteral reflux is backward flow of urine (or contrast medium) from the urinary bladder up to the kidney. It can be demonstrated on a cystogram or voiding cystourethrogram.
56. Cystogram
57. Voiding cystourethrogram
58. To remove gas and fecal material from the intestines so it doesn't obscure the urinary tract
59. The collection bag must always be placed lower than the urinary bladder to prevent retrograde flow of urine. The catheter should be clamped prior to administration of contrast medium to ensure adequate filling of the bladder. The clamp should be released following completion of the procedure or prior to the post-void film.
60. Start
61. 30°
62. Right
63. To enhance filling of the renal pelves, calyces, and proximal ureters
64. Water-soluble iodinated contrast medium
65. The use of tomography can help demonstrate the kidneys and ureters free of superimposition by gas and/or fecal material, and better visualize calculi, cysts, and tumors in the urinary tract.
66. The carbonation in the beverage fills the stomach with gas and pushes the intestines inferiorly, creating a radiolucent window through which the kidneys can be visualized.
67. Suspended respiration
68. 14 × 17 in.; iliac crest
69. Midway between the xiphoid process and iliac crests on the midsagittal plane
70. 70–75 kVp to produce high-contrast radiographs of the urinary tract

71. 40–60°
72. Left
73. Asymmetry of the obturator foramina and ischial spines
74. 5–20° caudad; 2 in. directly superior to the symphysis pubis
75.

Projection	CR Angle/ Angle of Part	Centering Point	Film Size	Structures Seen
AP urinary tract post-injection	CR = perpendicular part = 0°	Midsagittal plane at the level of the iliac crests	14 × 17 in. lw	Major and minor calyces, renal pelves, highlighted renal cortex and medullary tissue, ureters, and urinary bladder
LPO urinary bladder	CR = perpendicular (10° caudad when neck of bladder and proximal urethra of interest) part = 40–60°	2 in. superior to the symphysis pubis and 2 in. medial to plane passing through elevated ASIS	10 × 12 in. lw or cw	Urinary bladder, distal ureters (particularly right ureterovesical junction)
RPO urinary tract	CR = perpendicular part = 30°	Sagittal plane 3 in. medial to elevated ASIS at the level of the iliac crests	14 × 17 in. lw	Left kidney parallel to film plane, right kidney in profile, right ureter away from the spine; calyces, renal pelves, renal cortex and medullary tissue, and urinary bladder demonstrated

► ANSWER KEY FOR CROSSWORD PUZZLE

ACROSS

3. incontinence
6. hematuria
9. cystitis
10. uremia
11. nephrectomy
12. calyces
13. oliguria
14. hemodialysis
15. IVP
16. infraperitoneal
17. renalectopia

DOWN

1. micturition
2. nephroptosis
4. catheterization
5. nephrolith
7. urinalysis
8. anuria
9. cystoscope
11. nephron

► DISCUSSION OF ATYPICAL CASE STUDY

1. The discussion of the case study involving an intravenous urogram on the very tall hypersthenic male should include a review of many of the patient care tasks that are required of the radiologic technologist. How to move the patient appropriately, the questions to ask when obtaining a patient history, and how to evaluate contrast reactions are all subjects that should be addressed. Centering for the AP projection of the kidneys would be somewhat higher due to the patient's body type. The patient should be positioned in a 40–60° LPO to demonstrate the right ureterovesical junction.

DIGESTIVE SYSTEM 15

 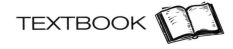

Objectives:

Following the completion of this chapter, the student will be able to:

1. Given diagrams or radiographs, name and describe the anatomy of the digestive system, to include the pharynx, esophagus, stomach, small intestine, and large intestine.
2. Discuss the orientation of the stomach according to body habitus, physical position, and respiration.
3. Identify the functions of each of the structures in the digestive system.
4. Outline the physiologic activities of digestion as they relate to each of the digestive organs.
5. Describe patient preparation and care relative to various radiographic examinations of the digestive system.
6. Discuss the use of contrast media in radiographic examinations of the digestive system, to include preferred type and route of administration.
7. List and describe the basic projections for examinations of the digestive system, to include preferred type and size of image receptor, central location, and structures best demonstrated.
8. Discuss the appropriate information to be obtained as part of the patient history in preparation for examinations of the digestive system.
9. Discuss the appropriate patient preparation for each of the examinations of the digestive system.
10. Practice positioning the basic projections of the digestive system on another student or phantom.
11. Describe the breathing instructions for radiographic examinations of the digestive system.
12. Describe equipment considerations and exposure factors relative to radiography of the digestive system.
13. Identify alternative methods for evaluating the digestive system.
14. State the criteria used to determine positioning accuracy on radiographs of the digestive system.
15. Evaluate radiographs of the digestive system in terms of positioning, centering, image quality, radiographic anatomy, and pathology.
16. Define terminology associated with the digestive system, to include anatomy, procedures, and pathology.

Chapter Outline

I. ANATOMY OF DIGESTIVE SYSTEM
   A. The Alimentary Canal
      1. mouth
      2. pharynx
      3. esophagus
      4. stomach
      5. small intestine
      6. large intestine
      7. appendix
      8. rectum
   B. Dimensional Anatomy
   C. Accessory Organs of Digestion
      1. liver
      2. gallbladder
      3. pancreas
II. PHYSIOLOGY OF THE DIGESTIVE SYSTEM
III. RELATED TERMINOLOGY
IV. PROCEDURAL CONSIDERATIONS
   A. Patient Preparation
   B. Room Preparation
   C. Positioning Considerations
   D. Alternate Procedures
      1. enteroclysis
      2. sialography
   E. Pediatric Imaging
   F. Breathing Instructions
   G. Exposure Factors
   H. Equipment Considerations
V. RADIOGRAPHIC POSITIONING
   A. Esophagus: AP, RAO, Lateral
      1. technical considerations
      2. shielding
      3. patient positioning
      4. part positioning
      5. central ray
      6. breathing instructions
      7. image evaluation
      8. critical anatomy
   B. UGI: PA, AP, RAO, Lateral, LPO Stomach
      1. technical considerations
      2. shielding
      3. patient positioning
      4. part positioning
      5. central ray
      6. breathing instructions

       7. image evaluation

       8. critical anatomy

   C. Small Bowel: PA/AP

      1. technical considerations

      2. shielding

      3. patient positioning

      4. part positioning

      5. central ray

      6. breathing instructions

      7. image evaluation

      8. critical anatomy

   D. Colon: AP/PA, RPO, LPO, AP Axial Rectosigmoid Region, Lateral Rectum, Lateral Decubitus

      1. technical considerations

      2. shielding

      3. patient positioning

      4. part positioning

      5. central ray

      6. breathing instructions

      7. image evaluation

      8. critical anatomy

 VI. SUMMARY

VII. CRITICAL THINKING & APPLICATION QUESTIONS

VIII. FILM CRITIQUE

SAMPLE 50-MINUTE LESSON ◄

PREPARATION STEP   ESTIMATED TIME—10 MINUTES

A. Assemble teaching aids
  1. Overhead projector
  2. Overhead transparencies
    a. included in *Instructor's Resource Manual*
  3. UGI and BE equipment
  4. Anatomic model
  5. Radiographs

B. Introduce topic of positioning of the digestive system. Lecture will include Chapter Objectives 8, 11, and 14.

C. Opening discussion
  1. Anatomy and procedural considerations have been presented. This lecture will continue with the positioning of the digestive system.
  2. The position/projections necessary to perform exams of the upper gastrointestinal system will be included in this lesson.
  3. The radiographic exams of the digestive system that we will discuss (except drinking esophagus) should be done on expiration. A grid should be used for the radiographs, and all children and adults of reproductive age should be shielded. Most fluoroscopy units project the radiation from under the table, so shield under the patient also.

PRESENTATION STEP

ESTIMATED TIME—40 MINUTES

TEACHING OUTLINE	TEACHING AIDS & METHODS
I. Examination Procedures for the Upper Gastrointestinal System	*Transparency of esophagus and stomach*
A. AP Esophagus	
1. technical considerations	
a. 14 × 17 in. film lengthwise	
2. positioning	*Radiographs of AP barium-filled esophagus*
a. supine position on table	
b. arms at sides, knees flexed	
c. upper edge of cassette 2–3 in. above top of shoulders	
3. central ray	
a. perpendicular to middle of cassette at T5–T6	
4. breathing instructions	
a. exposure made while patient swallowing barium	*Cup of barium with straw*
5. structures visualized	
a. barium-filled esophagus from pharynx to cardiac antrum	
B. RAO Esophagus	*Radiographs of RAO barium-filled esophagus*
1. technical considerations	
a. 14 × 17 in. film lengthwise	
2. positioning	
a. rotate patient to a 35–45° RAO position	
(1) hypersthenic 35°	
(2) asthenic 45°	
b. upper edge of cassette 2–3 in. above top of shoulders	
c. right edge of collimator light to right side of patient's spine	
3. central ray	
a. perpendicular to middle of cassette at T5–T6	
4. breathing instructions	
a. exposure made while patient swallowing barium	
5. structures visualized	
a. barium esophagus from pharynx to cardiac antrum	
C. Lateral Esophagus	*Radiographs of barium-filled esophagus lateral*
1. technical considerations	
a. 14 × 17 in. film lengthwise	
2. positioning	
a. right or left lateral	
b. upper edge of cassette 2–3 in. above top of shoulders	
3. central ray	
a. perpendicular to middle of cassette at T5–T6	
4. breathing instructions	
a. exposure made while patient swallowing barium	

 5. structures visualized
    a. barium-filled esophagus from pharynx to
       cardiac antrum
D. PA Stomach (UGI)   *PA stomach radiographs*
  1. technical considerations
    a. 11 × 14 in. film lengthwise
    b. 14 × 17 in. film lengthwise
    c. 10 × 12 in. film lengthwise
  2. positioning
    a. prone position on table
    b. midsagittal plane centered to table if use
       14 × 17 in. film
    c. center 1–2 in. away from spine over stomach
       if smaller film and patient is not asthenic
  3. central ray
    a. perpendicular to level of duodenal bulb
    b. sthenic: 1–2 in. above inferior margin of ribs
    c. hypersthenic: 3–4 in. above inferior margin of
       ribs
  4. structures visualized
    a. fundus, *barium-filled body,* greater and lesser   ***face down—barium down***
       curvature of stomach, duodenal bulb, and
       C-loop
E. AP Stomach (UGI)   *AP stomach radiographs*
  1. technical considerations
    a. 11 × 14 in. film lengthwise
    b. 14 × 17 in. film lengthwise
    c. 10 × 12 in. film lengthwise
    d. grid required
  2. positioning
    a. supine position on table
    b. midsagittal plane centered to table if use
       14 × 17 in. film
    c. center 1–2 in. away from spine over stomach
       if smaller film and patient is not asthenic
  3. central ray
    a. perpendicular to level of duodenal bulb
  4. structures visualized
    a. *barium-filled fundus,* body, greater and lesser   ***face up—barium up***
       curvature of stomach, duodenal bulb, and
       C-loop
F. RAO Stomach (UGI)   *RAO stomach radiographs*
  1. technical considerations
    a. 11 × 14 in. film lengthwise
    b. 10 × 12 in. film lengthwise
  2. positioning
    a. rotate patient to a 40–70° RAO position
       (1) asthenic 40°
       (2) hypersthenic 70°
  3. central ray
    a. perpendicular to level of duodenal bulb

  4. structures visualized
    a. pyloric canal and duodenal bulb   *face down—barium down*
    b. fundus, *barium-filled body,* greater and lesser
       curvature of stomach, duodenal bulb, and
       C-loop
  G. Lateral Stomach (UGI)   *Lateral stomach radiographs*
    1. technical considerations
      a. 11 × 14 in. film lengthwise
      b. 10 × 12 in. film lengthwise
    2. positioning
      a. right lateral position
    3. central ray
      a. perpendicular to level of duodenal bulb
      b. between the midcoronal plane and the anterior
         surface of abdomen
    4. structures visualized
      a. pyloric canal and duodenal bulb
      b. fundus, body, greater and lesser curvature of
         stomach, duodenal bulb, and C-loop,
         duodenojejunal junction
  H. LPO Stomach (UGI)   *LPO stomach radiographs*
    1. technical considerations
      a. 11 × 14 in. film lengthwise
      b. 10 × 12 in. film lengthwise
    2. positioning
      a. rotate patient to a 40–70° LPO position
    3. central ray
      a. perpendicular to level of duodenal bulb
    4. structures visualized
      a. pyloric canal and duodenal bulb
      b. *barium-filled fundus,* body, greater   *face up—barium up*
         and lesser curvature of stomach,
         duodenal bulb, and C-loop
  I. PA/AP Small Bowel   *small bowel radiographs*
    1. technical considerations
      a. 14 × 17 in. film lengthwise
      b. time marker indicating post-ingestion time
         should be included on film
    2. patient preparation
      a. patient drinks 8 oz more of barium
    3. positioning
      a. prone or supine
    4. central ray
      a. perpendicular to level of duodenal bulb for
         first film
      b. perpendicular to level of iliac crest for
         subsequent films
    5. structures visualized
      a. duodenum and jejunum on initial film
      b. jejunum and ileum on subsequent films

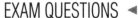

APPLICATION STEP   ESTIMATED TIME—2 HOURS

Study Assignment

A. Finish reading Chapter 15 in the text.
B. Complete Chapter 15 in the *Applications Manual.*
C. Be sure you can locate all the anatomy discussed on the anatomic model and on the appropriate radiograph.

TESTING STEP

Questions on this material will be included in exam given at end of this chapter.

EXAM QUESTIONS ◄

Multiple Choice

1. There normally is no advanced preparation necessary for which exam of the gastrointestinal system?
    A. esophagram
    B. UGI
    C. small bowel series
    D. barium enema

2. For which body habitus is it necessary to center 3–4 in. above the inferior margin of ribs for a radiograph of the stomach?
    A. hypersthenic
    B. sthenic
    C. hyposthenic
    D. asthenic

3. Which part of the small intestines is a retroperitoneal structure?
    A. ileocecal valve
    B. ileum
    C. jejunum
    D. duodenum

4. Name the parts of the colon beginning at the ileocecal valve and ending at the anus.
    A. cecum, ascending colon, splenic flexure, transverse colon, hepatic flexure, descending colon, sigmoid colon, rectum
    B. cecum, ascending colon, hepatic flexure, transverse colon, splenic flexure, descending colon, sigmoid colon, rectum
    C. cecum, descending colon, splenic flexure, transverse colon, hepatic flexure, ascending colon, sigmoid colon, rectum
    D. cecum, descending colon, hepatic flexure, transverse colon, splenic flexure, ascending colon, sigmoid colon, rectum

5. What part of the colon is responsible for creating the haustra?
   A. rugae
   B. anal sphincter
   C. teniae coli
   D. mesocolon

6. What anatomical part of which organ is situated in the curve of the duodenum or C-loop?
   A. tail of the pancreas
   B. head of the pancreas
   C. pyloric antrum of the stomach
   D. body of the stomach

7. What is the term used to describe inflammation of the sacs or pouches protruding outward from the wall of the alimentary canal?
   A. Crohn's disease
   B. appendectomy
   C. colitis
   D. diverticulitis

8. What name is given to an abnormal sessile or pedunculated growth that extends into the lumen of the alimentary canal?
   A. intussusception
   B. rectocele
   C. imperforate anus
   D. polyp

9. What is the usual patient preparation for an UGI?
   A. no advance preparation is necessary
   B. the patient should refrain from eating breakfast on the morning of the exam but can drink clear liquids
   C. the patient should not eat or drink anything for at least 8 hours before the exam
   D. the patient should be NPO from midnight the day of the exam and perform a cleansing enema the evening before the exam

10. Under what conditions should the patient be instructed to contact his/her personal physician following an exam where they received barium either orally or rectally?
    1. no bowel movement within 24 hours after the examination
    2. abdominal distension
    3. rectal bleeding
       A. 1 only
       B. 1 and 2 only
       C. 2 and 3 only
       D. 1, 2, and 3

11. How is the salivary duct dilated for injection of contrast media?
    A. the patient is asked to suck on a lemon
    B. the duct is anesthetized and a cannula is inserted
    C. the patient is asked to puff out the cheeks
    D. the patient is asked to bear down as if to have a bowel movement

12. The special breathing technique(s) used to increase the intrathoracic and intra-abdominal pressures is (are) called the:

    1. Valsalva maneuver

    2. Mueller maneuver

    3. Schuller maneuver

    A. 1 only

    B. 1 and 2 only

    C. 2 and 3 only

    D. 1, 2, and 3

13. What optimal kVp range should be used when performing double-contrast study of the alimentary canal?

    A. 70–75 kVp

    B. 85–90 kVp

    C. 100–105 kVp

    D. 115–120 kVp

14. Which of the following positions would visualize barium in the body of the stomach?

    A. RAO stomach

    B. LPO stomach

    C. AP stomach

    D. lateral esophagus

15. Which barium enema position demonstrates the splenic flexure and the descending colon?

    A. LPO

    B. RAO

    C. RPO

    D. left lateral

ANSWER KEY

1. A	4. B	7. D	10. D	13. B
2. A	5. C	8. D	11. A	14. A
3. D	6. B	9. C	12. B	15. C

APPLICATIONS MANUAL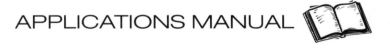

ANSWER KEY FOR STUDY QUESTIONS ◄

1. Alimentary canal
2. Teeth, tongue, salivary glands, liver, gallbladder, and pancreas
3. Mucosa
4. Buccal
5. Roof of the oral cavity
6. The tongue functions to move and direct food in the mouth posteriorly toward the pharynx.
7. Mastication
8. Fauces
9. Soft

10. Parotid
11. They tear and grind the food into smaller pieces that can mix more easily with saliva.
12. Submandibular (submaxillary), sublingual, and parotid
13. Swallowing
14. Anterior to the submandibular (submaxillary) under the tongue
15. The epiglottis covers the opening to the larynx so that food passes posteriorly down the laryngopharynx and into the esophagus.
16. 10 in. (25 cm)
17. 6th cervical; 11th thoracic
18. The esophagus transports food and fluids from the pharynx to the stomach.
19. Esophageal hiatus; 10th thoracic
20. Cardiac antrum
21. 11th thoracic
22. Rugae
23. Cardiac
24. Chyme
25. Fundus, body, and pyloric antrum (pylorus)
26. Pyloric
27. Fundus
28. It acts as a valve at the pyloric orifice to adjust the flow of chyme into the duodenum.
29. Greater curvature
30. Angular
31. The characteristic J-shape of the stomach becomes very elongated on an asthenic patient. Also, the stomach is situated lower and closer to the spine than in the sthenic abdomen.
32. Superiorly
33. Large intestine
34. Duodenum, jejunum, and ileum
35. Ileum
36. Left upper quadrant
37. Ileum
38. Duodenum
39. Right lower quadrant
40. Plicae circularis
41. Jejunum
42. Cecum
43. Vermiform process; right lower quadrant
44. On the left upper and lower quadrants of the abdomen, extending between the splenic flexure and the sigmoid colon
45. Sigmoid colon
46. Right colic (hepatic) flexure
47. Rectal ampulla
48. Teniae coli
49. The left colic (splenic) flexure
50. Haustra
51. The liver is an accessory organ because it manufactures bile, which aids in the digestion of fats.
52. Duodenum
53. It produces pancreatic juice, which contains digestive enzymes. These enzymes break down proteins, carbohydrates, and fats in food.
54. When a bolus of food passes from the mouth into the oropharynx, the epiglottis closes off the trachea so that the bolus can continue through the laryngopharynx and into the esophagus. Since the opening to the trachea is covered by the epiglottis, air cannot be inhaled or exhaled.
55. Peristalsis
56. Enzymes
57. Small intestine
58. Defecation

59. 3–5 hours
60. 24 hours
61. Feces
62. Esophagus
63. Small intestine
64. The different preparations are a direct result of the different functions performed by the esophagus and stomach. Because foods and fluids travel through the esophagus quickly after being swallowed, there is no advanced preparation. However, the stomach acts as a holding chamber so that food does not pass rapidly into the small intestine. Because the stomach should be empty for an upper GI exam, patients should be instructed to refrain from eating or drinking anything for at least 8 hours prior to the exam.
65. Barium sulfate is administered rectally as the positive agent. Room air is generally used as the negative contrast agent and is also administered rectally.
66. Sialography
67. Enterocylsis
68. Suspended expiration
69. Take in a deep breath, hold the breath in, and bear down as if trying to move the bowels.
70. T5–6
71. Respiration is temporarily suspended for 1–3 seconds during swallowing.
72. 35–45°; more
73. To help in demonstrating esophageal reflux and/or a diaphragmatic hernia by increasing the intrathoracic and intra-abdominal pressure
74. Midcoronal plane or midaxillary line
75. RAO
76. Duodenal bulb; 2nd lumbar
77. The central ray must be directed higher than on the sthenic patient to the level of L-1, about 3–4 in. above the inferior margin of the ribs.
78. Barium sulfate (because it is located posteriorly)
79. 40–70°
80. More
81. Lateral
82. AP or PA
83. RAO
84. The spine should appear lateral; the posterior aspect of the lower ribs should be superimposed.
85. Midway between the vertebral column and left lateral margin of the thorax
86. It indicates the amount of time that has elapsed since ingestion of the contrast medium. Since this is a functional study, the time it takes for the contrast medium to pass through the small intestine and into the large intestine will be noted by the radiologist.
87. When barium sulfate passes through the terminal ileum into the cecum
88. The iliac crests
89. Air; barium sulfate
90. Posteriorly
91. LPO or RAO
92. 35–45°
93. It is obtained prior to fluoroscopy to assess bowel obstruction, patient preparation, and the presence of radiopaque stones.
94. 30–45° cephalad; ASIS
95. The plicae circularis are more numerous in the jejunum and are coated by the barium sulfate, giving it a more feathery appearance. Since they are not as predominant in the ileum, this part of the small intestine appears much smoother.
96. LPO or RAO
97. Right lateral decubitus
98. Lateral
99. The soft tissue depression just above the greater trochanters

100.

Projection	CR Angle/ Angle of Part	Centering Point	Film Size	Structures Seen
RAO esophagus	CR = 0° part = 35–45°	Level of T5–6	14 × 17 in. lw	Barium-filled esophagus from lower pharynx to cardiac antrum—esophagus should be demonstrated between spine and heart
Right lateral	CR = 0° part = 90°	Level of the duodenal bulb (L-2 on sthenic patient)	10 × 12 in. lw	Pyloric canal and duodenal bulb are well demonstrated; fundus, body, greater and lesser curvatures of stomach, C-loop of duodenum, and proximal jejunum are also demonstrated.
RPO large intestine	CR = 0° part = 35–45°	Level of the iliac crests	14 × 17 in. lw	Entire large intestine, particularly the splenic flexure and descending colon
Left lateral rectum	CR = 0° part = 90°	Level of soft tissue depression above the greater trochanter	10 × 12 in. lw or 11 × 14 in. lw	Rectosigmoid area is demonstrated; rectum is demonstrated in profile; sigmoid colon is also demonstrated.

WORD SEARCH

```
B  U  F  E  G  A  S  T  R  I  T  I  S  X  N
L  S  W  L  V  S  N  T  T  Q  Y  R  D  O  D
W  N  A  U  S  E  A  T  M  M  N  A  I  D  B
D  V  O  L  V  U  L  U  S  R  W  T  O  E  N
S  I  T  I  C  I  D  N  E  P  P  A  H  X  J
V  P  V  K  T  I  I  C  O  E  O  T  R  P  G
W  O  M  E  I  A  L  X  C  M  K  X  R  J  S
C  Q  Y  U  R  U  P  S  K  B  G  O  O  J  M
V  R  C  S  M  T  U  I  D  X  C  G  M  E  F
O  A  O  W  M  S  I  P  T  T  I  L  E  U  S
I  W  L  H  S  B  K  C  O  S  S  F  H  Y  H
L  A  I  U  N  T  D  C  U  L  N  O  G  A  C
B  D  T  L  S  S  E  V  Q  L  Y  O  Y  W  M
P  N  I  N  F  L  A  T  U  S  A  P  C  Y  F
I  K  S  L  E  T  I  Z  S  D  U  H  S  E  E
```

WORD LIST:

1. APPENDICITIS
2. COLITIS
3. CONSTIPATION
4. CROHNS
5. DIVERTICULA
6. FLATUS
7. GASTRITIS
8. HEMORRHOIDS
9. ILEUS
10. INTUSSUSCEPTION
11. MUMPS
12. NAUSEA
13. POLYPS
14. PROCTOCELE
15. ULCER
16. VOLVULUS

▶ DISCUSSION OF ATYPICAL CASE STUDIES

1. This would be an excellent case study to assign as a project. The 2-week-old baby brought to the imaging department by his parents for an esophagram would need to be immobilized on a octagon or papoose board. Due to the age of this child it may be necessary to provide a heat lamp so he will not get too cold. There would be no special preparation for this exam of the esophagus. The child should be shielded underneath for the fluoroscopy. If barium is used as a contrast medium, it could be given through a feeding tube connected to a syringe. The feeding tube then could be put through a nipple, which the child would have in his mouth. The barium could be regulated by pushing on the plunger of the syringe. The child could also drink the barium from a bottle. The barium would stay in the blind pouch of the esophagus and most likely need to be aspirated by the use of a feeding tube and syringe. There are several different types of esophageal atresia, however, that may be imaged differently.

2. The axial projection of the sigmoid could easily be performed on the patient with the colostomy who is unable to lie in a prone position. The CR would be directed 30–45° cephalad to the level of the ASIS if a 14 × 17 in. film is used and 2 in. inferior to the level of the ASIS if a 11 × 14 in. film is used. Care must be taken not to injure the stoma when the cone-shaped tip or catheter with an inflatable cuff is inserted. Gloves must be worn by the radiographer when removing a dressing or drainage pouch.

BILIARY SYSTEM 16

 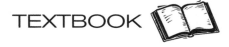

Objectives:

Following the completion of this chapter, the student will be able to:

1. Given diagrams or radiographs, name and describe the anatomy of the biliary system, to include the liver, gallbladder, and ducts.
2. Discuss the orientation of the gallbladder according to body habitus, physical position, and respiration.
3. Identify the functions of each of the structures in the biliary system.
4. Discuss the production and movement of bile in the biliary system.
5. Identify the main vascular structures associated with the liver.
6. Define cholelith and discuss its appearance radiographically.
7. Describe the relationship of the pancreas with the biliary system.
8. Describe patient preparation and care relative to various radiographic examinations of the biliary system.
9. Describe room preparation and identify the supplies needed for examinations of the biliary system.
10. Discuss the use of contrast media in radiographic examinations of the biliary system, to include type and route of administration.
11. List and describe the basic projections for examinations of the biliary system, to include preferred type and size of image receptor, central ray location, and structures best demonstrated.
12. Discuss the appropriate information to be obtained as part of the patient history in preparation for examinations of the biliary system.
13. Practice positioning the basic projections of the biliary system on another student or phantom.
14. Describe the breathing instructions for radiographic examinations of the biliary system.
15. Describe equipment considerations and exposure factors relative to radiography of the biliary system.
16. Identify alternative methods for evaluating the biliary system.
17. Define terminology associated with the biliary system, to include anatomy, procedures, and pathology.
18. State the criteria used to determine positioning accuracy on radiographs of the biliary system.
19. Evaluate radiographs of the biliary system in terms of positioning, centering, image quality, radiographic anatomy, and pathology.

Chapter Outline

I. ANATOMY OF THE BILIARY SYSTEM
  A. Liver
  B. Gallbladder
    1. choleliths
  C. Biliary Ducts
II. PHYSIOLOGY OF THE BILIARY SYSTEM
III. ANATOMY & PHYSIOLOGY OF THE PANCREAS
IV. RELATED TERMINOLOGY
V. PROCEDURAL CONSIDERATIONS
  A. Oral Cholecystography
    1. patient preparation
    2. room preparation
    3. positioning considerations
  B. Cholangiography
    1. operative cholangiogram
    2. t-tube cholangiogram
    3. percutaneous transhepatic cholangiography (PTC)
  C. Endoscopic Retrograde Cholangiopancreatogram (ERCP)
    1. patient preparation
    2. room preparation
    3. positioning considerations
  D. Breathing Instructions
  E. Exposure Factors
  F. Equipment Considerations
VI. RADIOGRAPHIC POSITIONING
  A. Cholecystogram: PA, LAO
    1. technical considerations
    2. shielding
    3. patient positioning
    4. part positioning
    5. central ray
    6. breathing instructions
    7. image evaluation
    8. critical anatomy
VII. SUMMARY
VIII. CRITICAL THINKING & APPLICATION QUESTIONS
IX. FILM CRITIQUE

▶ SAMPLE 50-MINUTE LESSON

PREPARATION STEP	ESTIMATED TIME—10 MINUTES

A. Assemble teaching aids
  1. Overhead projector
  2. Overhead transparencies
    a. included in *Instructor's Resource Manual*

3. skeleton
4. radiographs
B. Introduce topic of the anatomy of the biliary system. Lecture will include Chapter Objectives 1 to 7.
C. Opening discussion
1. The gallbladder is not imaged in the x-ray department very often due to the ability of ultrasound to visualize this organ. It takes a radiologic exam, however, to visualize if the gallbladder is working.
2. The biliary ducts are also visualized in a variety of ways using radiation. You may be called to surgery to take a radiograph after the gallbladder has been removed, as these surgeries are quite common.
3. It is important to learn the anatomy of the biliary system well as this will promote a better understanding of the imaging procedures we will discuss later.

PRESENTATION STEP   ESTIMATED TIME—40 MINUTES

TEACHING OUTLINE	TEACHING AIDS & METHODS
I. Anatomy of the Biliary System	*Transparency of system*

I. Anatomy of the Biliary System
   A. Refers to Structures Concerned With the Production, Storage, and Movement of Bile
   B. Liver
      1. body's largest solid organ
      2. two major lobes
         a. right
         b. left
      3. two minor lobes
         a. caudate
            (1) posterior to right lobe
         b. quadrate
            (1) inferior surface
      4. parenchyma
         a. functional unit of liver
      5. highly vascular
         a. hepatic artery
         b. portal vein
      6. produces bile
      7. many other functions
   C. Gallbladder
      1. located in shallow depression on the posteroinferior surface of liver
      2. bottom lies approximately at level of ninth costal cartilage
      3. position dependent on
         a. body type
            (1) hypersthenic: higher, more transverse, more lateral
            (2) asthenic: low and close to spine
         b. body position
         c. respiration
      4. fundus, body, neck
      5. stores and concentrates bile
         a. choleliths

Pass around gallstones

            (1) may form when bile becomes too concentrated

        (2) 80% formed from combination of
        calcium, cholesterol, bile pigments
         (a) radiolucent   *Gallstone x-ray*
         (b) radiopaque
       (3) high-risk group
        (a) women
           (i) over 40
           (ii) overweight
           (iii) pregnant
           (iv) taking oral contraceptives

  D. Biliary Ducts
    1. transports bile through system
    2. right and left hepatic ducts   *Draw ducts on board*
      a. drain bile from major lobes of liver
    3. common hepatic duct
      a. distal to where hepatic ducts unite
    4. cystic duct
      a. extend from the gallbladder
    5. common bile duct
      a. distal to joining of common hepatic duct and
      cystic duct
      b. hepatopancreatic ampulla
        (1) distended portion proximal to sphincter
      c. enters duodenum through hepatopancreatic
      sphincter
    6. pancreatic duct
      a. extends from pancreas
      b. converges with common bile duct
      c. hepatopancreatic ampulla
        (1) distended portion proximal to sphincter
      d. enters duodenum through hepatopancreatic
      sphincter

II. Physiology of Biliary System
  A. When Chyme Enters Duodenum, Cells Secrete
  Cholecystokinin, Which Prompts Gallbladder to
  Contract and Expel Bile and the Pancreas to
  Secrete Pancreatic Juices
    1. bile emulsifies fats
    2. pancreatic juice breaks down protein,
    carbohydrates, and fats

III. Pancreas
  A. Not Part of Biliary System
  B. Accessory Organ of Digestion
  C. Behind Stomach
  D. Retroperitoneal
  E. Head, Body, Tail
  F. Head Situated in "C" Loop
  G. Tail in Hilum of Spleen
  H. Endocrine Gland—1%
    1. ductless pancreatic islets
  I. Exocrine Gland—99%
    1. pancreatic duct

IV. Related Terminology
  A. Important to Learn Terms
    1. chole: bile
    2. cholangio: bile duct

3. cholecysto: bile sac (gallbladder)
4. hepato: liver

APPLICATION STEP

ESTIMATED TIME—2 HOURS

Study Assignment

A. Begin reading Chapter 16 in the text.
B. Begin Chapter 16 in the *Applications Manual*.
C. Be sure you can locate where the gallbladder is located in patients of various body habitus, body positions, and respiration.

TESTING STEP

Questions on this material will be included in exam given at end of this chapter.

EXAM QUESTIONS

Multiple Choice

1. Which substance in the body emulsifies fats, is produced in the liver, and is stored in the gallbladder?
   A. water
   B. bile
   C. cholecystokinin
   D. cholesterol

2. A radiographic exam done specifically to visualize the gallbladder is termed
   A. cholecystopaque
   B. cholangiography
   C. cholecystography
   D. cystography

3. Where would the gallbladder be located on a hypersthenic individual?
   A. lower and nearer the spine than in a sthenic individual
   B. higher and more lateral than in a sthenic individual
   C. lower and more lateral than in a sthenic individual
   D. higher and nearer the spine than in a sthenic individual

4. The patient with which body habitus would need to be obliqued more steeply for an LAO radiograph of the gallbladder?
   A. hypersthenic
   B. sthenic
   C. hyposthenic
   D. asthenic

5. What is the purpose of giving a patient a "fatty meal" as part of a routine oral cholecystogram?
   A. it causes the gallbladder to expand for better visualization
   B. it causes the contrast to stay in the gallbladder longer
   C. it causes the gallbladder to contract
   D. it causes the pancreas to stop releasing its secretions

6. Which population is at highest risk for forming gallstones?
   1. women over 40
   2. overweight men over 40
   3. women who are pregnant or taking oral contraceptives
      A. 1 only
      B. 2 only
      C. 1 and 3 only
      D. 1 and 2 only

7. On an abdomen radiograph, gallstones composed primarily of cholesterol and bile pigments would be
   A. visible when the gallbladder is *not* filled with contrast only
   B. visible when the gallbladder is filled with contrast only
   C. visible before the gallbladder is filled with contrast, and visible after the gallbladder is filled with contrast
   D. *not* visible before the gallbladder is filled with contrast, and *not* visible after the gallbladder is filled with contrast

8. What is the name of the hormone secreted by the intestinal mucosa after ingesting food that prompts the gallbladder to contract and expel bile?
   A. cholecystokinin
   B. cholecystopaque
   C. choledochus
   D. cholesteremia

9. Which position visualizes stratification of gallstones during an oral cholecystogram?
   A. LAO
   B. LPO
   C. recumbent lateral
   D. right lateral decubitus

10. What is the purpose of performing an operative cholangiogram?
    A. to visualize the bile ducts to evaluate patency
    B. to visualize the bile ducts before they are surgically removed
    C. to visualize the gallbladder contracting
    D. to visualize gallstones within the gallbladder

11. Which exam of the biliary ducts is accomplished by inserting a long needle through the liver directly into the bile duct?
    A. operative cholangiography
    B. T-tube cholangiography
    C. percutaneous transhepatic cholangiography
    D. endoscopic retrograde cholangiopancreatography

12. For which exam is a fiberoptic endoscope passed through the mouth to the hepatopancreatic ampulla by a gastroenterologist?
    A. operative cholangiography
    B. T-tube cholangiography
    C. percutaneous transhepatic cholangiography
    D. endoscopic retrograde cholangiopancreatography

13. How is the location of the gallbladder affected when the patient takes in a deep inspiration?
   A. it does not move
   B. it moves 1–3 in. inferiorly
   C. it moves 1–3 in. superiorly
   D. it moves 1–3 in. medially

14. Why is it necessary for the patient to be in an oblique position when a radiograph of the gallbladder is performed?
   A. to move the gallbladder away from the spine
   B. to place the gallbladder closer to the image receptor
   C. to visualize stratification of any gallstones
   D. to better evaluate the biliary ducts

15. Which kVp range is recommended for all radiography of the biliary system to enhance subject contrast?
   A. 50–60 kVp
   B. 65–75 kVp
   C. 80–90 kVp
   D. 95–105 kVp

ANSWER KEY

1. B	4. D	7. B	10. A	13. B
2. C	5. C	8. A	11. C	14. A
3. B	6. C	9. D	12. D	15. A

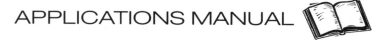

APPLICATIONS MANUAL

ANSWER KEY FOR STUDY QUESTIONS

1. Liver, gallbladder, and bile ducts
2. Right
3. Immediately under the right hemidiaphragm
4. Four
5. Falciform ligament
6. Hepatocytes
7. Microscopic functional unit of the liver that is hexagon-shaped and located in the parenchyma of the liver
8. Canaliculi
9. Porta hepatis
10. Emulsification of fats, which enables them to be absorbed and digested
11. Caudate and quadrate
12. Liver
13. Posteroinferior
14. Ninth
15. Fundus, body, and neck
16. Higher; laterally
17. Anterior
18. To store and concentrate bile

19. It has muscular walls.
20. Fundus
21. Cystic
22. Gallstone
23. Right and left hepatic
24. Cystic duct and common hepatic duct
25. Cholecystokinin
26. Hepatopancreatic ampulla
27. Breakdown of large lipid (fat) globules into smaller particles that can be more readily digested and absorbed
28. The nipplelike projections of the common bile duct into the lumen of the duodenum
29. The head of the pancreas is situated in the C-loop of the duodenum
30. Glucagon and insulin
31. Tail
32. Cholecystography
33. Cholangiography
34. A fatty meal preparation administered orally to the patient to evaluate the contracting ability of the gallbladder; it is not a contrast medium.
35. Vomiting and diarrhea may result in a poorly visualized gallbladder.
36. Cholecystopaque
37. PA upright or right lateral decubitus projections
38. More
39. To demonstrate the patency of the ducts, look for residual stones, and evaluate the status of the hepatopancreatic sphincter.
40. An endoscopic retrograde cholangiopancreatogram is a procedure used to diagnose biliary and pancreatic pathologic conditions.
41. Sterile procedure is followed to prevent infection since a needle is inserted through the skin and liver and directly into the bile ducts. Universal precautions are followed since the radiographer and radiologist may be exposed to blood and body fluids (eg, bile).
42. Suspended expiration
43. 15–40° (depending upon body habitus)
44. Lower costal margin
45. False; the pancreas is not an organ in the biliary system.
46. True
47. True
48. False; the liver continuously manufactures bile.
49. False; the position of the gallbladder is affected by body habitus, respiration, and physical position (supine vs upright).

50.

Projection	CR Angle/ Angle of Part	Centering Point	Film Size	Structures Seen
PA upright gallbladder	CR = perpendicular part = 0° prone	Approx. 1 in. lower than the lower costal margin since the GB drops down when a person stands upright	10 × 12 in. lw	Fundus, body, and neck of the gallbladder
LAO gallbladder	CR = perpendicular part = 15–40° depending upon body habitus	Lower costal margin	10 × 12 in. lw	Fundus, body, and neck of the gallbladder
Right lateral decubitus gallbladder	CR = horizontal part = 90°	Lower costal margin	10 × 12 in. cw	Fundus, body, and neck of the gallbladder

▶ ANSWER KEY FOR CROSSWORD PUZZLE

ACROSS

1. cystic duct
5. ERCP
6. hepatomegaly
7. cholangitis
8. fundus
10. gallstone
11. cholecystectomy
13. lithotripsy
15. emulsification
16. hepatocyte

DOWN

1. chole
2. cirrhosis
3. hepatitis
4. jaundice
7. cholecystopaque
9. acholia
10. gallbladder
12. liver
14. bile

▶ DISCUSSION OF ATYPICAL CASE STUDY

1. This patient has had to be rescheduled from the previous day because her gallbladder did not visualize. This has occurred because she vomited following ingestion of the contrast medium pills. The gallbladder should be visible on today's exam because she did not vomit following ingestion of the contrast medium. As this woman has an asthenic body habitus, her gallbladder is lower and closer to the spine. She should be rotated more (about 40°) for the LAO position because of this. If she is unable to stand for an upright radiograph, a right lateral decubitus can be substituted. The purpose of both the upright and right lateral decubitus radiographs is to see stratification of gallstones.

MAMMOGRAPHY 17

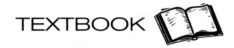

TEXTBOOK

Objectives:

Following the completion of this chapter, the student will be able to:

1. Given diagrams or radiographs, name and describe the anatomy of the breast.
2. Describe the relationship of the structures of the breast to the thorax.
3. Define terminology associated with breast imaging, to include anatomy, procedures, and pathology of both the male and female breast.
4. Describe the patient preparation and care relative to the radiographic examination of the breast.
5. Describe the basic and recommended routine projections of the breast.
6. Describe the guidelines for labeling radiographs of the breast.
7. Discuss alternate projections of the breast for demonstrating "hard to demonstrate" lesions.
8. Identify the breathing instructions for radiographic examination of the breast.
9. Practice positioning basic projections of the breast using teaching aids or another student or appropriate subject.
10. Describe procedural modifications for patients who have unusual body habitus or physical limitation.
11. State the criteria used to determine positioning accuracy on radiographs of the breast.
12. Evaluate radiographs of the breast in terms of positioning, centering, image quality, radiographic anatomy, and pathology.
13. Discuss how imaging the augmented breast differs from imaging the natural breast tissue.
14. Describe the process of needle localization for biopsy procedures.
15. Describe the procedure for imaging breast biopsy specimens.
16. Explain how other imaging modalities compliment the mammographic examination.
17. Describe equipment considerations and exposure factors relative to radiography of the breast.
18. Explain the importance of critical quality assurance and control related to breast imaging.

Chapter Outline

  I. ANATOMY OF THE BREAST
    A. Breast Pathology
  II. RELATED TERMINOLOGY
  III. PROCEDURAL CONSIDERATIONS
    A. Patient Preparation
    B. Room Preparation
    C. Positioning Considerations

     D. Alternate Projections/Procedures

     E. Breathing Instructions

     F. Exposure Factors

     G. Equipment Considerations

     H. Image Processing

IV. RADIOGRAPHIC POSITIONING

     A. Craniocaudal (CC) Projection, Mediolateral (MLO) Projection

       1. patient positioning

       2. part positioning

       3. central ray

       4. image evaluation

       5. critical anatomy

V. SUPPLEMENTARY PROJECTIONS

     A. Caudocranial

     B. Tangential

     C. Roll—Medial or Lateral

     D. Exaggerated CC

     E. Cleavage

     F. Spot Compression

     G. Magnification

VI. VARIATIONS ON MAMMOGRAPHY

     A. Augmented Breast Mammography

     B. Galactography

     C. Needle Localization for Biopsy

     D. Specimen Imaging

VII. ANCILLARY & COMPLIMENTARY MODALITIES

     A. Magnetic Resonance Imaging

     B. Digital Mammography

     C. Other Developing Breast Imaging Techniques

VIII. SUMMARY

IX. CRITICAL THINKING & APPLICATION QUESTIONS

X. FILM CRITIQUE

► SAMPLE 50 MINUTE LESSON

PREPARATION STEP   ESTIMATED TIME—10 MINUTES

     A. Assemble teaching aids

       1. Overhead projector

       2. Overhead transparencies

         a. included in *Instructor's Resource Manual*

       3. Mammograms

     B. Introduce topic of anatomy of the breast. Lecture will include Chapter Objectives 1 to 3.

     C. Opening discussion

       1. One in every eight women will develop breast cancer in her lifetime. A woman's best defense is a monthly breast self-exam (BSE), clinical examination by her physician, and the mammogram.

2. This chapter will provide mammography content at an entry level for the student radiographer. Several additional requirements are needed to become specialized in this area of radiography.

3. Mammograms are hung on the viewbox in the same orientation as they were taken. A right lateral projection of the breast is displayed on the viewbox in the same orientation as if we were looking at the patient's right breast in the unit under compression. This is different from regular radiography.

4. It is important to know the basic anatomy of the breast to obtain the most diagnostic mammogram possible.

PRESENTATION STEP   ESTIMATED TIME—40 MINUTES

TEACHING OUTLINE	TEACHING AIDS & METHODS
I. Anatomy of the Breast	
A. Male breast	
1. rudimentary and without function	
2. although rare, can also have breast cancer	
B. Female breast	*Transparency of anatomy of breast*
1. accessory reproductive organ	
2. modified sweat gland specialized to secrete milk during lactation	
3. develop in response to estrogen and progesterone, which is produced in the ovaries	
C. Location	
1. overlie the pectoralis major muscles	
2. extend from the 2nd to 7th rib and from sternum to axilla	
3. "tail" of breast extends up to axilla	
a. tail of Spence	
D. Components of the Normal Breast	*Mammograms*
1. inframammary crease	
a. junction at inferior part of breast and anterior chest wall	
2. retromammary space	
a. layer of fat between fibrous tissue covering pectoralis major muscle and fibrous tissue around posterior portion of breast	
3. nipple	
a. area where the ducts collect into opening	
4. areola	
a. pigmented area surrounding nipple	
E. Composition of the Normal Breast	
1. 15–20 glandular lobes	
a. more located superiorly and laterally in breast	
b. each lobe divided into many lobules	
2. lobule	
a. basic structural unit of the breast	
b. composed of acini	
(1) secreting units during lactation	
c. functional unit of the breast	
(1) terminal ductal lobular unit (TDLU)	
(a) drains from 10–100 acini	

        d. draining ducts
          (1) lactiferous ductules
          (2) lactiferous ducts
             (a) eight or more open into nipple
        e. decrease in size and number with age and following pregnancy
          (1) involution
    3. cooper's (suspensory) ligament
        a. provides support for the breast connective tissue, which forms dense strands
        b. lose elasticity around the age of 50
    4. lymphatic vessels
        a. drain laterally into axillary lymph nodes (75%)
        b. drain medially into internal mammary nodes behind sternum

F. Types of Breasts
    1. important to obtain accurate patient history to provide appropriate exposure factors for type of breast
    2. age, parity, and hormones affect density of the breast
    3. fibroglandular   *Examples on mammogram*
        a. most dense type of breast
          (1) requires more radiographic exposure
        b. post-puberty to 30 years
          (1) later if nulliparous
        c. pregnant and lactating
    4. fibroglandular fatty
        a. breast has about equal fat to fibrous tissue
          (1) requires less radiographic exposure than fibroglandular
        b. 30–50 years
          (1) may change to this type of breast at younger age if have had several pregnancies
        c. post-menopausal women on hormone replacement
    5. fatty
        a. males
        b. post menopausal
        c. fat replaces fibrous tissue
          (1) requires least amount of radiographic exposure
        d. very little contrast on mammogram

G. Breast Mobility
    1. the breast has some mobility at the lateral and inferior margins
        a. elevating the breast from the inframammary crease upward allows for more effective compression on the CC projection
        b. the lateral mobility allows the radiographer to position the cassette parallel to the pectoralis muscle and enhance compression of MLO projection

2. the mobile part of the breast should be placed on the immobile part of the unit and the immobile part of the breast should be placed against the movable compression device
   a. will obtain maximum breast tissue on radiograph
H. Breast Pathology   *Examples on mammogram*
   1. mammography images many abnormalities
      a. changes in symmetry of breast tissue densities
      b. architectural or ductal patterns
      c. contour or skin thickening
      d. masses
      e. calcifications
      f. dilation of veins or ducts
      g. fibrocystic changes in the breast
   2. important for radiographer to recognize demonstrable pathology and then relate symptoms and history to positioning and technical factors

APPLICATION STEP   ESTIMATED TIME—2 HOURS

Study Assignment

A. Begin reading Chapter 17 in the text.
B. Begin Chapter 17 in the *Applications Manual*.
C. Read the atypical case study in Chapter 17 of the *Applications Manual* and research how the mammogram described could be accomplished.

TESTING STEP

Questions on this material will be included in exam given at end of this chapter.

EXAM QUESTIONS ◄

Multiple Choice

1. Which type of individual would exhibit fibroglandular fatty breasts?
   1. a woman who is breast feeding
   2. a woman between the ages of 30 and 50
   3. a woman under 30 who has had several children
      A. 1 only
      B. 1 and 2 only
      C. 2 and 3 only
      D. 1, 2, and 3

2. Which type of individual would exhibit fatty breasts?
   1. a 25-year-old male
   2. a post-menopausal woman who is 55

3. a post-menopausal woman on hormonal replacement who is 60

   A. 1 only

   B. 1 and 2 only

   C. 2 and 3 only

   D. 1, 2, and 3

3. Which breast tissue type requires the highest amount of radiographic exposure?

   A. fibroglandular

   B. fibroglandular fatty

   C. fatty

   D. the male breast

4. Which margin(s) of the breast have some mobility?

   1. superior margin

   2. lateral margin

   3. inferior margin

      A. 1 only

      B. 1 and 2 only

      C. 2 and 3 only

      D. 1, 2, and 3

5. Which of the following breast pathologies or conditions can be demonstrated on a mammogram?

   1. dilation of veins or ducts

   2. calcifications

   3. skin thickening

      A. 1 and 2 only

      B. 2 and 3 only

      C. 1 and 3 only

      D. 1, 2, and 3

6. What is the average glandular dose for the *four* standard projections in a screening mammogram?

   A. 0.1 rad

   B. 0.4 rad

   C. 1.5 rad

   D. 3 rad

7. What name is given to the benign tumor that develops from epithelial and fibroblastic tissue brought on by higher than normal estrogen levels in women under 30?

   A. fibroadenoma

   B. fibrocystic disease

   C. cysts

   D. carcinoma

8. Which projections are normally obtained when performing a screening mammogram?

   A. caudocranial and lateromedial oblique

   B. exaggerated craniocaudad and exaggerated caudocranial

   C. craniocaudad and mediolateral oblique

   D. 90° mediolateral and 90° lateromedial

9. The radiographic exam that demonstrates the collecting ducts surrounding the nipple by injecting contrast media into them through the orifice is called
   A. needle localization
   B. breast scintigraphy
   C. fine-needle aspiration
   D. galactography

10. What is the appropriate kVp range for mammography?
   A. 5–10 kVp
   B. 15–20 kVp
   C. 25–30 kVp
   D. 35–40 kVp

11. When using AEC in mammography, which part of the breast should be over the photocell selected?
   A. the nipple and areola
   B. the anterior third
   C. the middle third
   D. the posterior third

12. It is recommended that AEC NOT be used for which type of breast?
   A. augmented
   B. fibroglandular
   C. fibroglandular fatty
   D. fatty

13. The pectoralis major muscle should be demonstrated down to the level of the nipple for which projection?
   A. craniocaudal
   B. caudocranial
   C. mediolateral oblique
   D. exaggerated craniocaudal

14. What is (are) the purpose(s) of using breast compression?
   1. it minimizes superimposition
   2. it helps the patient take in a deep breath
   3. it immobilizes the patient
      A. 2 only
      B. 3 only
      C. 1 and 2 only
      D. 1 and 3 only

15. Where would 3 o'clock be located on a woman's left breast?
   A. superior
   B. inferior
   C. medial
   D. lateral

ANSWER KEY

1. B	4. C	7. A	10. C	13. C
2. B	5. D	8. C	11. B	14. D
3. A	6. B	9. D	12. A	15. D

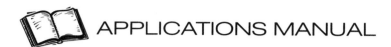 APPLICATIONS MANUAL

▶ ANSWER KEY FOR STUDY QUESTIONS

1. Mammography
2. The female breast serves as an accessory reproductive organ whose purpose is to secrete milk for the nourishment of offspring.
3. Pectoralis major; 2nd; 7th
4. Areola
5. Inframammary crease
6. Upper outer
7. The axillary tail extends toward the axillary lymph nodes. This contact with the lymphatic system makes an excellent transport mechanism for cancer cells to spread to different regions of the body.
8. 15–20
9. Suspensory (Cooper's) ligaments
10. Fibroglandular
11. Fatty; because she is post-menopausal and has had several pregnancies, glandular tissue has atrophied and been replaced by fatty breast tissue.
12. Fibroglandular fatty
13. Fibroglandular
14. Declining hormone levels from the hysterectomy probably resulted in less glandular and more fatty breast tissue; however, the hormone replacement therapy does cause the breast tissue to become somewhat denser, resembling the breast tissue of a younger person.
15. Inclusion of the pectoralis major muscle signifies that all of the breast tissue was demonstrated on the radiograph.
16. It causes it to become more dense and harder to penetrate.
17. The answer is yes for items A–E as all of them can be demonstrated on a mammogram.
18. The lateral and inferior margins are more mobile than the medial and superior margins.
19. Mastectomy
20. Nulliparous; multiparous
21. Lumpectomy
22. Microcalcifications
23. MSQA is the Mammography Quality Standards Act, which is legislation passed in Congress in October 1994 to improve and standardize optimum quality of mammography.
24. .03
25. 35–40
26. After age 50
27. Components of deodorants, perfumes, and powders (i.e., aluminum flakes) may cause unwanted artifacts on the resultant breast images that may be mistaken for unfortunate pathologic conditions.
28. Quadrant method and clock method
29. Craniocaudad (CC) and mediolateral oblique (MLO)
30. Lower outer
31. 30–70°

32. The angle of the C-arm should match the angle of the patient's pectoralis major muscle. Very thin patients generally require a greater angle than overweight patients.

33. Generally, when the breast is correctly positioned the nipple is in profile. This is important so that the nipple is not mistaken for a lesion.

34. 25–35 lbs

35. FB refers to from below since the C-arm is rotated 180° to place the x-ray tube below the breast and the cassette holder at the most superior aspect of the breast

36. The true 90° mediolateral (ML) or lateromedial (LM) projection is used to verify a finding that may be demonstrated on the routine projections. To localize a lesion in the breast, a 90° degree ML or LM projection can demonstrate whether the lesion is in the medial or lateral aspect of the breast.

37. The breast tissue is rolled so that previously superimposed tissues in the craniocaudad (CC) projection do not appear in the same region.

38. Superior; inferior

39. When the most medial tissue of both breasts must be demonstrated

40. Galactography

41. Magnification projections are recommended when there is a need to evaluate calcifications or architectural detail within the breast.

42. A needle localization procedure is performed to obtain a core sample or fine-needle aspiration of cells for biopsy. It is also performed to localize a lesion that is usually nonpalpable immediately prior to surgical excision.

43. A total of four projections are taken on each breast: CC and MLO with the prosthesis in place using light compression, and CC and MLO with the prosthesis displaced against the chest wall using regular compression.

44. It is a specialized piece of equipment used for needle localization procedures. Stereotactic capabilities allow for localizing a lesion in three dimensions with greater precision and accuracy.

45. 25–30

46. The appropriate photocell should be selected for the size of the breast being imaged and placed under the densest portion of the breast.

47. Molybdenum

48. The x-ray tube is positioned so that the cathode is over the chest wall, directing the best part of the beam through the thicker breast tissue adjacent to the pectoralis region.

49. Compression flattens and separates breast structures, minimizing superimposition; it improves visibility of detail since tissue thickness is decreased; radiographic exposure is reduced due to decreased tissue thickness; it helps the patient hold still, reducing motion artifacts; and it produces a more uniform density.

50. Weekly

WORD SEARCH

```
N O I T A C I F I N G A M G V
T L S V Q R Y T S I B S E A W
R M I L U A Q O I N I R D L U
D O T E C N E P S F O L I A T
T F I N O I S S E R P M O C P
Q L T F P O B S H A S I L T H
M L S I A C Y D T M Y M A O S
Q U A D R A N T S M S S T G A
B X M C I U T C O A L O E R A
I Q E D T D U N R R W L R A E
P C C U Y A S J P Y P R A M T
V R E S D D T P P P D U L F J
P H O B Q V P I I N K O L N S
G C R G D P G N O L J Y T L M
A R A F C X W F W N F C Q M J
```

WORD LIST

1. AREOLA
2. BIOPSY
3. COMPRESSION
4. CRANIOCAUDAD
5. GALACTOGRAM
6. LACTATION
7. MAGNIFICATION
8. MASTITIS
9. MEDIOLATERAL
10. NIPPLE
11. PARITY
12. PROSTHESIS
13. QUADRANT
14. SPOT
15. TAIL OF SPENCE

► DISCUSSION OF ATYPICAL CASE STUDY

1. This is another case study that may take a little research on the part of the students. If the woman who was paralyzed from the waist down could not sit in a wheelchair for the mammogram, she could remain on the stretcher. The CC projection could be accomplished by leaving her in the supine position and positioning the breast so that the lateral side of the film holder would be against her chest. The projection would be a caudocranial rather than the routine craniocaudal. She would need to roll on her side for the lateral projections. The film holder would be placed against her sternum and a lateromedial projection could be obtained. The fact that this woman has very little breast tissue would add to the difficulty of doing this exam. If there was concern that there was not enough tissue over the AEC, a manual technique can be employed. If it is difficult to position her breast, a spatula can help pull the breast tissue into the correct location.

CARDIOVASCULAR SYSTEM 18

TEXTBOOK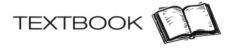

Objectives:

Following the completion of this chapter, the student will be able to:

1. Identify the major components of the cardiovascular system, to include their location and function.
2. Differentiate between pulmonary and systemic circulation.
3. Discriminate between veins and arteries with regard to size, location, and blood flow.
4. Define the term *angiography* and discuss its need in examinations of the cardiovascular system.
5. Discuss what is meant by an "interventional" procedure.
6. Describe the Seldinger technique, to include purpose, steps, and common access sites.
7. Discuss pre- and post-procedural patient care for an angiographic procedure.
8. Identify the indications for performing various angiographic procedures, including lymphangiography.
9. List and describe the equipment commonly used for angiographic procedures.
10. Define terminology associated with the cardiovascular system and special radiographic procedures, to include anatomy and pathology.
11. Discuss the relationship between the cardiovascular and lymphatic systems.

Chapter Outline

I. ANATOMY OF THE CARDIOVASCULAR SYSTEM
   A. Systemic Circulation
   B. Pulmonary Circulation
II. LYMPHATIC SYSTEM
III. RELATED TERMINOLOGY
IV. PROCEDURAL CONSIDERATIONS
   A. Diagnostic Procedures
   B. Therapeutic Procedures
V. PATIENT CARE
   A. Preparation
   B. Catheterization
   C. Post-procedural Care
VI. EQUIPMENT CONSIDERATIONS
   A. Guidewires and Catheters
   B. Contrast Media

  C. Imaging Equipment

  D. Automatic Injector

  E. Digital Subtraction Angiography (DSA)

VII. ANGIOGRAPHIC PROCEDURES

  A. Cardiac Catheterization and Coronary Angiography

  B. Interventions in the Cardiac Catheterization Lab

   1. percutaneous transluminal coronary angioplasty (PTCA)

   2. directional coronary atherectomy (DCA)

   3. coronary stents

   4. percutaneous transluminal coronary rotational ablation (PTCA) or rotoblator

   5. transluminal extraction (TEC)

  C. Cerebral Angiography

  D. Aortography

  E. Abdominal Angiography

  F. Selective Visceral Angiography

  G. Pulmonary Angiography

  H. Femoral Angiogram

  I. Upper Extremity Angiogram

  J. Venography

VIII. LYMPHANGIOGRAPHY

IX. SUMMARY

X. CRITICAL THINKING & APPLICATION QUESTIONS

► SAMPLE 50-MINUTE LESSON

PREPARATION STEP   ESTIMATED TIME—10 MINUTES

A. Assemble teaching aids

 1. Overhead projector

 2. Overhead transparencies

  a. included in *Instructor's Resource Manual*

 3. Model of heart

 4. Radiographs

B. Introduce topic of anatomy of the circulatory system

C. Opening discussion

 1. The anatomy presented should be a review of material learned in anatomy and physiology class. This information will aid you in your study of diagnostic and therapeutic procedures, which are presented in this chapter. This lesson will cover Objectives 1 to 4.

 2. You most likely will not be performing the angiographic procedures as a student or new technologist, but you will be radiographing patients who have undergone these procedures.

 3. You will spend some time in angiography observing and helping perform these exams, so this information will be very useful.

 4. Some of your careers will lead to angiography or cardiography, so learning these basic facts will be very helpful.

PRESENTATION STEP   **ESTIMATED TIME—40 MINUTES**

TEACHING OUTLINE	TEACHING AIDS & METHODS

I. Circulatory System

    A. Cardiovascular System

    B. Lymphatic System

II. Cardiovascular System

    A. Systemic Circulation

       1. begins with left ventricle

       2. includes all circulation except lungs

       3. complete circuit of blood through body takes only 23 seconds or 27 heartbeats

       4. arteries

          a. carry oxygenated blood from heart

          b. tunica intima

          c. tunica media

          d. tunica externa/adventitia

       5. arterioles

       6. capillaries

          a. where exchange of oxygen and nutrients occurs

          b. waste products filtered out

       7. venules

       8. veins

          a. carry deoxygenated blood to right atrium

          b. pressure in venous system lower than arterial system

          c. valves prevent backflow of blood

          d. tunica intima

          e. tunica media

          f. tunica externa/adventitia

             (1) walls not as thick, however

    B. Pulmonary Circulation

       1. delivers blood to the lungs

       2. deoxygenated blood pumped from right ventricle through right and left pulmonary arteries to lungs

       3. carbon dioxide exchanged for oxygen in lungs

       4. oxygenated blood transported through four pulmonary veins to left atrium

III. Lymphatic System

    A. Lymph Vessels

    B. Lymph Nodes

    C. Organs

       1. tonsils

       2. thymus gland

       3. spleen

    D. Filters Cellular Waste Products From Blood

    E. Helps Ward off Infections

    F. Fluid Leaks out of Capillaries Into Interstitial Space and Passes Through Permeable Membrane Into Lymphatic Vessels

       1. lymph

Teaching Aids & Methods notes:

Transparencies of systems (aligned with I. Circulatory System)

Transparency of arteries and veins (aligned with 4. arteries)

Reinforce that pulmonary arteries are only arteries in body carrying deoxygenated blood and pulmonary veins are only veins to carry oxygenated blood (aligned with B. Pulmonary Circulation)

Transparency of system (aligned with III. Lymphatic System)

    G. Lymph Vessels Have Valves so Fluid Flows to Heart

    H. Lymph Fluid Transported in Vessels to Lymph Nodes Clustered Throughout Body

    I. Lymph Nodes Filter out Bacteria and Destroy Pathogens to Help Cleanse Blood

    J. Lymph Vessels Drain Into Right Lymphatic Duct or Thoracic Duct, Which Both Drain Into the Subclavian Veins

IV. Procedural Considerations

    A. Angiography

       1. study of vessels of the body

    B. Diagnostic Procedures

       1. assessing vessel of interest using Seldinger technique

         a. catheter is threaded over guidewire to the site   *Examples of catheter and guidewires*

       2. water-soluble iodinated contrast medium injected with rapid filming of vessels

       3. image obtained through use of cinefluoroscopy or rapid film changers

       4. angiographic exams performed for

         a. aneurysms

         b. arteriovenous malformations

         c. stenoses

         d. evaluation of injury to vascular system

    C. Therapeutic Procedures

       1. use of angiographic procedure for treatment of patient

       2. thrombolytics

         a. streptokinase and urokinase

           (1) dissolve arterial blood clots

       3. insertion of inferior vena cava filters

         a. traps clots from deep vein thromboses before get to lungs

           (1) pulmonary emboli

       4. embolism therapy

         a. used to control or stop bleeding or cause infarction of vascular tumor

           (1) gelatin sponge

           (2) metallic coils

           (3) detachable balloons

           (4) alcohol

       5. stents

         a. used to restore normal blood flow to area

         b. stainless-steel tube mounted on angioplasty balloon

         c. used in

           (1) aorta

           (2) renal, subclavian, iliac, femoral arteries

           (3) biliary tree

APPLICATION STEP

Study Assignment

A. Begin reading Chapter 18 in the text.
B. Begin Chapter 18 in the *Applications Manual.*
C. Review the anatomy and physiology of the circulatory system in your anatomy and physiology book.

TESTING STEP

Questions on this material will be included in exam given at end of this chapter.

EXAM QUESTIONS ◄

Multiple Choice

1. The outer layer of the arteries and veins is named the
    A. tunica intima
    B. tunica media
    C. tunica adventitia
    D. cortex

2. The lymphatic system is a component of the cardiovascular system.
    A. true
    B. false

3. A weak area in a vessel's wall that causes it to balloon outward is a/an
    A. anastomosis
    B. aneurysm
    C. embolism
    D. phlebolith

4. An accumulation of clotted blood that leaks out of a blood vessel as the result of an injury is a/an
    A. arteriotomy
    B. aneurysm
    C. hematoma
    D. infarct

5. What name is given to the medications used to dissolve arterial blood clots?
    A. embolism
    B. thromboses
    C. angina
    D. thrombolytics

6. What is the purpose of vena cava filters?
    A. to filter out bacteria in the vena cava before it can enter the heart
    B. to restore normal blood flow to the heart
    C. to embolize the vena cava if there is excess bleeding
    D. to trap emboli from deep vein thromboses before they enter the lungs

7. The procedure in which a catheter is introduced directly into one of the chambers of heart to record hemodynamic and physiologic information is
   A. cardiac catheterization
   B. coronary angiography
   C. percutaneous transluminal coronary angioplasty
   D. digital subtraction angiography

8. The most common vessel used to access the coronary vessels for coronary angiography is the
   A. femoral vein
   B. femoral artery
   C. superior vena cava
   D. aortic arch

9. The radiographic exam done to rule out deep vein thrombosis is
   A. lower leg venogram
   B. upper extremity venogram
   C. popliteal arteriography
   D. vena cava venography

10. What is the purpose of the blue dye that is injected between the patient's toes during a lymphangiogram?
    A. localization of the lymph vessels
    B. opacification of the lymph vessels
    C. visualization of the lymph nodes
    D. visualization of the lymph vessels

11. Lymphangiogram radiographs taken 24 hours post-injection visualize the
    A. capillary beds
    B. arterioles and venules
    C. lymph vessels
    D. lymph nodes

12. The type of contrast commonly used to visualize the cardiovascular system is
    A. thin barium
    B. ethiodol
    C. water-soluble iodine
    D. oil-based iodine

13. Manual or mechanical pressure must be applied to the incision site following a procedure for a minimum of
    A. 5 minutes
    B. 10 minutes
    C. 20 minutes
    D. 30 minutes

14. Which interventional study actually removes plaque from the coronary artery by using a high-speed burr covered with diamond crystals?
    A. percutaneous transluminal coronary angioplasty (PTCA)
    B. directional coronary atherectomy (DCA)
    C. coronary stent placement
    D. percutaneous transluminal coronary rotational ablation (PTCRA)

15. Which diagnostic exam visualizes the blood supply to the brain?

    A. cerebral angiography

    B. aortography

    C. brachial angiography

    D. superior mesenteric arteriography

ANSWER KEY

1. C	4. C	7. A	10. A	13. B
2. B	5. D	8. B	11. D	14. D
3. B	6. D	9. A	12. C	15. A

APPLICATIONS MANUAL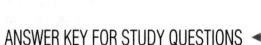

ANSWER KEY FOR STUDY QUESTIONS ◄

1. Cardiovascular; lymphatic

2. Arteries

3. Veins

4. Capillaries are located throughout the body's tissues. They consist of thin, semi-permeable walls through which these materials can pass.

5. About 23 seconds (27 heartbeats)

6. A. tunica intima

   B. tunica media

   C. tunica externa (adventitia)

7. Systemic

8. The pulmonary arteries are the only arteries to carry deoxygenated blood, whereas the pulmonary veins are the only veins in the body to carry oxygenated blood.

9. Venules

10. The contraction of skeletal muscles in the walls of the veins provides enough force to propel the blood to the heart.

11. They prevent the backflow of blood.

12. Right ventricle; left atrium

13. Angiography

14. The lymphatic system functions to filter cellular waste products from the blood, return interstitial fluid to the bloodstream, and help the body ward off infections.

15. Any three of the following:

    A. tonsils,

    B. thymus gland,

    C. spleen,

    D. lymph nodes,

    E. red bone marrow

16. Cardiology

17. A thrombus is a blood clot that forms in a vessel, partially or completely occluding it. An embolism is a blood clot or other foreign material (ie, fat or air bubble) that moves away from its site of formation, suddenly occluding an artery and obstructing the flow of blood to the tissues.

18. Any of the following: injury to vascular system (trauma), vascular tumor, AV malformation, stenosis of vessel

19. Thrombolytics

20. Vena cava filters are often used when patients have developed clots in their venous system, particularly deep vein thromboses in the lower extremities, and anticoagulation therapy is contraindicated. The filter will serve to trap clots before they can travel to the lungs or elsewhere in the body.

21. Embolization therapy is performed to stop bleeding in the case of excess hemorrhage from trauma or to cut off the blood supply to a vascular tumor prior to surgical excision. An embolization agent is administered during an angiogram once the source of the bleeding or vascular tumor has been identified. Blood will adhere to the agent, forming a clot that should control or stop the bleeding.

22. Any of the following: gelatin sponge (Gelfoam), metallic coils, detachable balloon, alcohol

23. The restore normal blood flow to an area by maintaining patency of the vessel supplying blood to the area

24. The stainless-steel stent is mounted on an angioplasty balloon catheter. The catheter is guided through the vessel to the area of interest, with the stent placed across the specific area of stenosis. Once the stent is in place, the balloon is inflated and the stent deployed, forcing the stent into the wall of the vessel. The balloon is deflated and the catheter removed, leaving the stent in place.

25. An explanation of the procedure, the reason it is needed, possible complications, and alternative procedures

26. The patient should be NPO for 6–8 hours prior to the procedure.

27. Common femoral artery in the groin area

28. Seldinger technique

29. To achieve hemostasis

30. 24

31. The catheter is used to deliver contrast media and other devices to a specific location inside the body. If one was not used, the contrast medium would be diluted by the time it reached the area of interest.

32. They help in engaging different blood vessels; the vessel of interest can be selected for examination.

33. Either ionic or nonionic iodinated contrast medium

34. To examine the blood vessels of the entire lower limb, the table must shift the patient to several different positions over the film changers.

35. Guidewires are required for the safe insertion, position, reposition, and exchange of catheters.

36. The pressure injector permits the contrast medium to be delivered in a controlled manner over a specific time, giving a specific amount at the correct flow rate. Since arterial blood flows rapidly, hand injection will not put enough contrast medium in the vessel rapidly enough, allowing it to become diluted.

37. Digital subtraction angiography (DSA)

38. Tricuspid; mitral

39. Left anterior descending; circumflex

40. Indication

41. Percutaneous transluminal coronary angioplasty (PTCA)

42. Directional coronary atherectomy (DCA) and transluminal extraction (TEC)

43. Right and left carotid arteries, right and left vertebral arteries

44. 4th lumbar

45. Hepatic, splenic, and left gastric

46. The circulation of the small intestine (except duodenum), the cecum, ascending colon, and the transverse colon

47. To visualize the circulation, perfusion, and function of the kidney, and to demonstrate the exact location of the renal artery supplying the kidney

48. Femoral vein, inferior vena cava, right atrium, tricuspid valve, right ventricle, pulmonary trunk, left pulmonary artery

49. In the case of unexplained peripheral swelling, lymphangiography may be helpful in demonstrating a possible obstruction of the lymph vessels or nodes.

50. Since lymph is clear, the lymphatic vessels are difficult to find for cannulation. The blue indicator dye will cause the lymphatic vessels in the foot to visualize. A cutdown procedure is performed on the dorsum of the foot to insert a needle in the vessel for injection of contrast medium. A film is taken 24 hours after the completion of injection to demonstrate the lymph nodes.

ANSWER KEY FOR CROSSWORD PUZZLE ◄

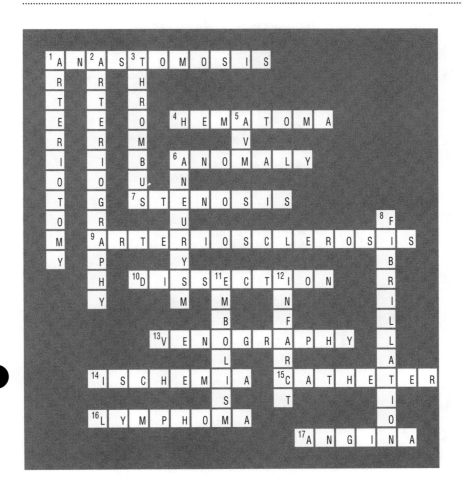

ACROSS

1. anastomosis
4. hematoma
6. anomaly
7. stenosis
9. arteriosclerosis
10. dissection
13. venography
14. ischemia
15. catheter
16. lymphoma
17. angina

DOWN

1. arteriotomy
2. arteriography
3. thrombus
5. AVM
6. aneurysm
8. fibrillation
11. embolism
12. infarct

ATYPICAL CASE STUDY DISCUSSION ◄

1. Communication with the anxious hearing-impaired patient will be in writing. The patient should be given as much time as necessary to write down any questions he may have. Prearranged hand signals should be used during the exam to ascertain if the patient is doing all right and for any other necessary directions. Care must be taken that the patient feel that he has not been forgotten as he will not be able to hear what is going on around him. Eye contact is very important and written explanations should be given if it becomes necessary during the exam.

3

SECTION

▶ TRANSPARENCY MASTERS

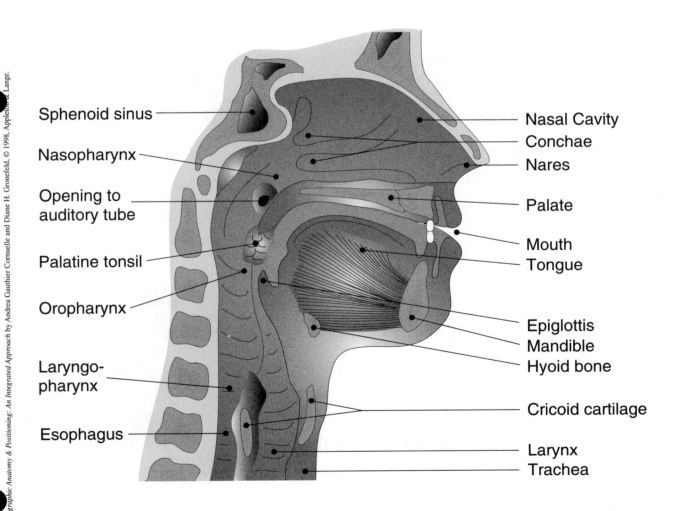

Superior

Sagittal plane through head and neck

Anterior

Nasopharynx
Oropharynx
Laryngopharynx

Sphenoid sinus

Nasopharynx

Opening to auditory tube

Palatine tonsil

Oropharynx

Laryngo-pharynx

Esophagus

Nasal Cavity
Conchae
Nares

Palate

Mouth
Tongue

Epiglottis
Mandible
Hyoid bone

Cricoid cartilage

Larynx
Trachea

Figure 2–2.

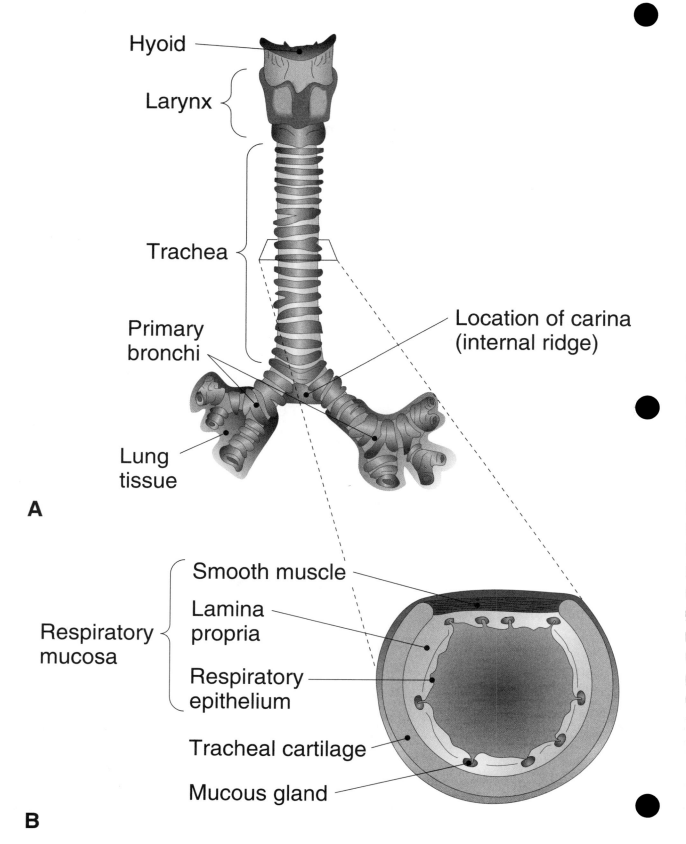

Hyoid

Larynx

Trachea

Primary
bronchi

Lung
tissue

Location of carina
(internal ridge)

A

Smooth muscle

Lamina
propria

Respiratory
mucosa

Respiratory
epithelium

Tracheal cartilage

Mucous gland

B

Figure 2–4A, B.

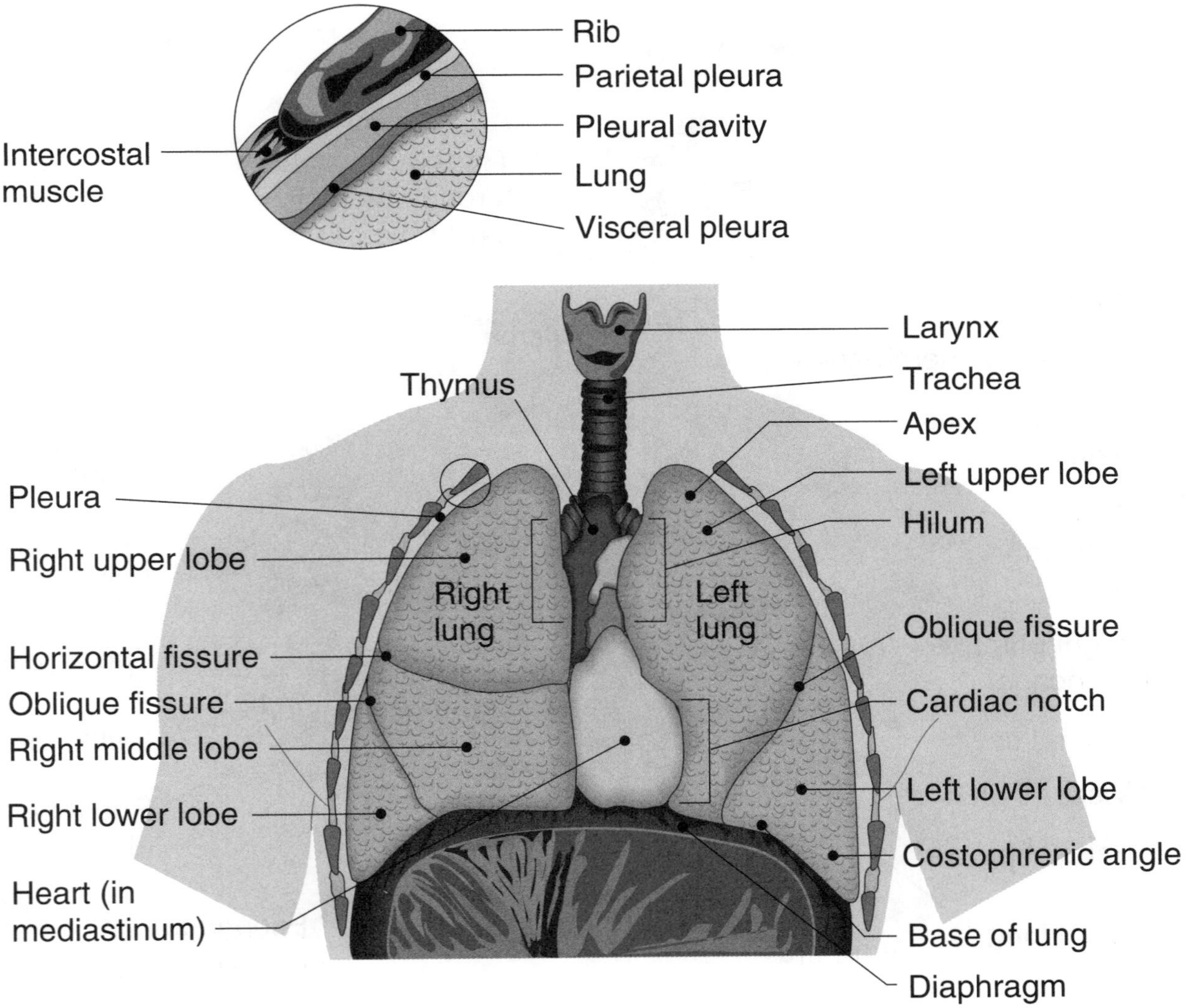

Rib
Parietal pleura
Pleural cavity
Lung
Visceral pleura
Intercostal muscle

Thymus
Larynx
Trachea
Apex
Left upper lobe
Hilum
Pleura
Right upper lobe
Right lung
Left lung
Oblique fissure
Horizontal fissure
Oblique fissure
Cardiac notch
Right middle lobe
Right lower lobe
Left lower lobe
Costophrenic angle
Heart (in mediastinum)
Base of lung
Diaphragm

Figure 2–7.

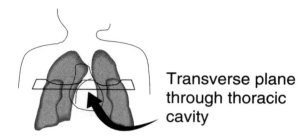

Transverse plane
through thoracic
cavity

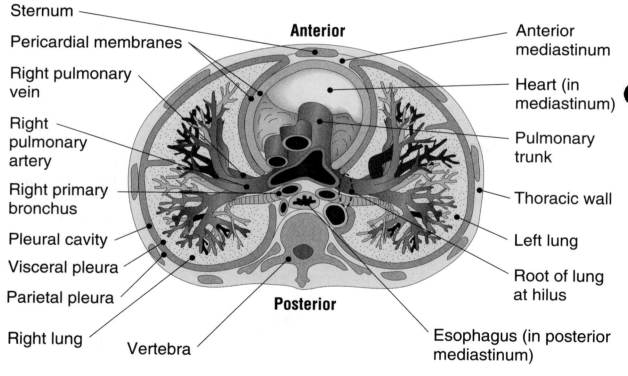

Sternum

Pericardial membranes

Right pulmonary
vein

Right
pulmonary
artery

Right primary
bronchus

Pleural cavity

Visceral pleura

Parietal pleura

Right lung

Vertebra

Anterior

Posterior

Anterior
mediastinum

Heart (in
mediastinum)

Pulmonary
trunk

Thoracic wall

Left lung

Root of lung
at hilus

Esophagus (in posterior
mediastinum)

Figure 2–8.

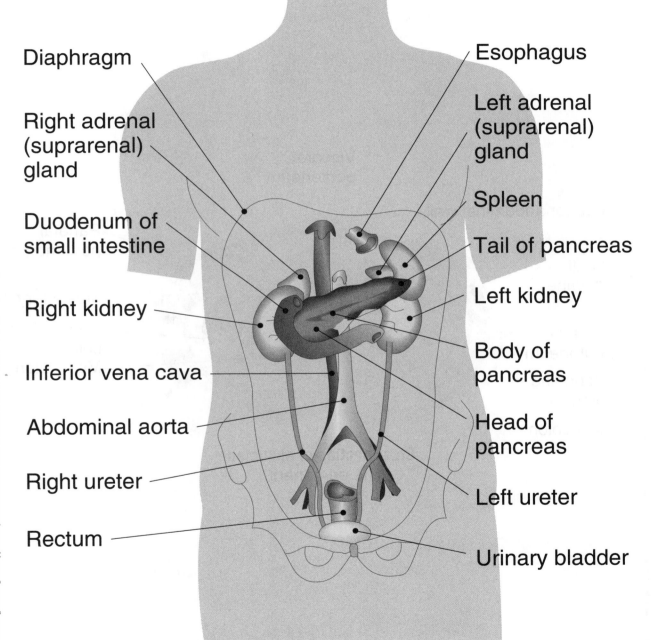

Diaphragm

Right adrenal
(suprarenal)
gland

Duodenum of
small intestine

Right kidney

Inferior vena cava

Abdominal aorta

Right ureter

Rectum

Esophagus

Left adrenal
(suprarenal)
gland

Spleen

Tail of pancreas

Left kidney

Body of
pancreas

Head of
pancreas

Left ureter

Urinary bladder

Figure 3–1.

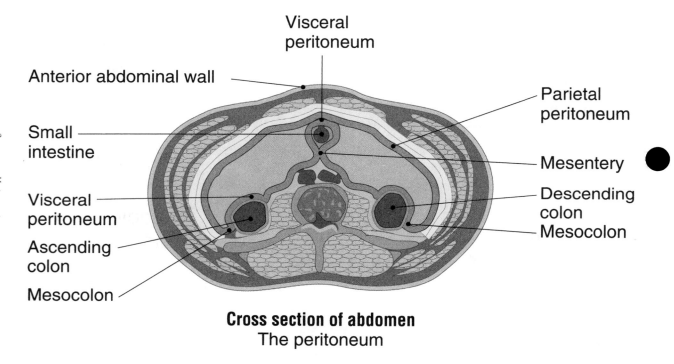

Cross section of abdomen
The peritoneum

Figure 3–3.

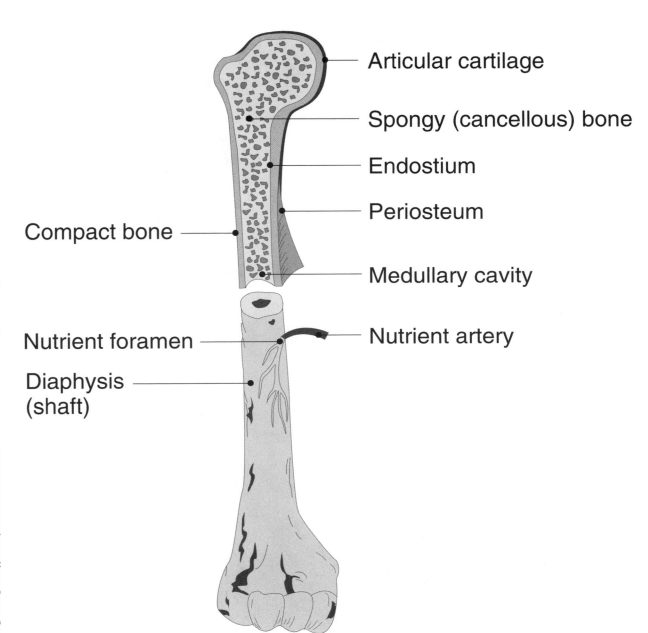

Articular cartilage

Spongy (cancellous) bone

Endostium

Periosteum

Compact bone

Medullary cavity

Nutrient foramen

Nutrient artery

Diaphysis
(shaft)

Figure 4–3.

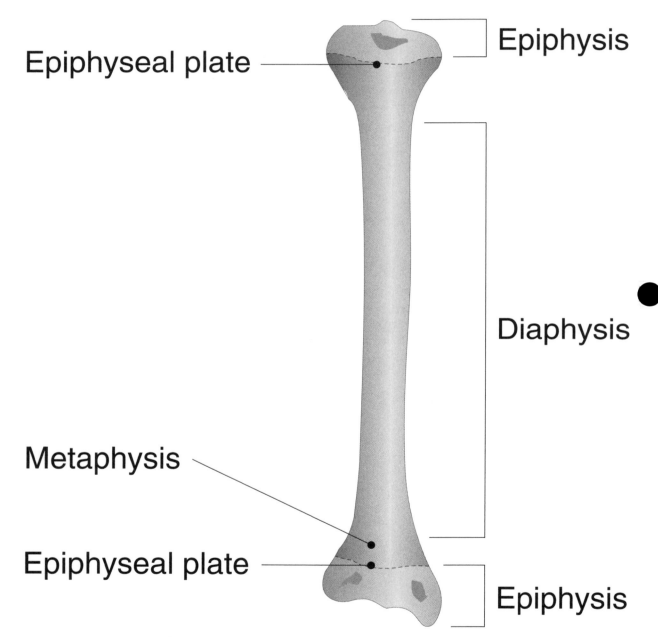

Epiphyseal plate

Epiphysis

Diaphysis

Metaphysis

Epiphyseal plate

Epiphysis

Figure 4–7.

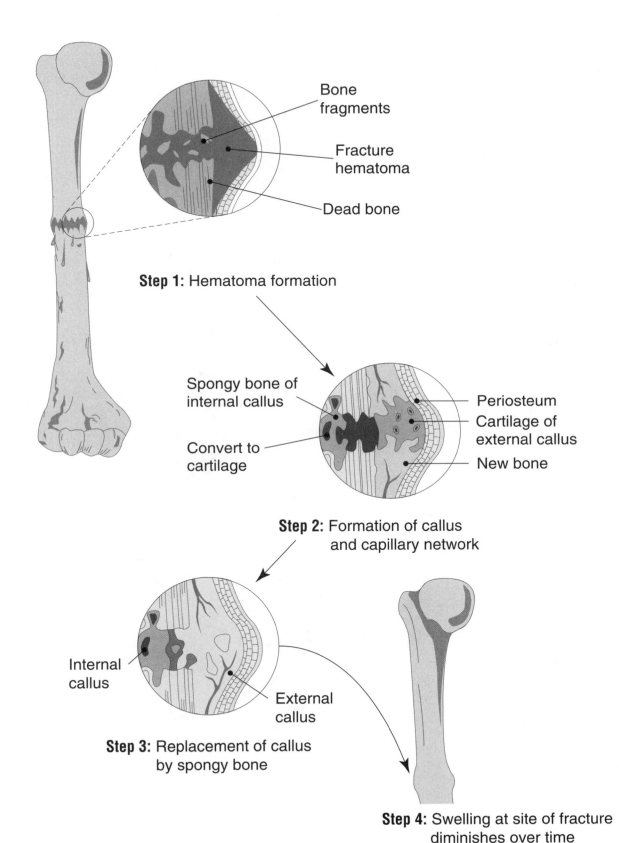

Bone
fragments

Fracture
hematoma

Dead bone

Step 1: Hematoma formation

Spongy bone of
internal callus

Convert to
cartilage

Periosteum

Cartilage of
external callus

New bone

Step 2: Formation of callus
and capillary network

Internal
callus

External
callus

Step 3: Replacement of callus
by spongy bone

Step 4: Swelling at site of fracture
diminishes over time

Figure 4–9.

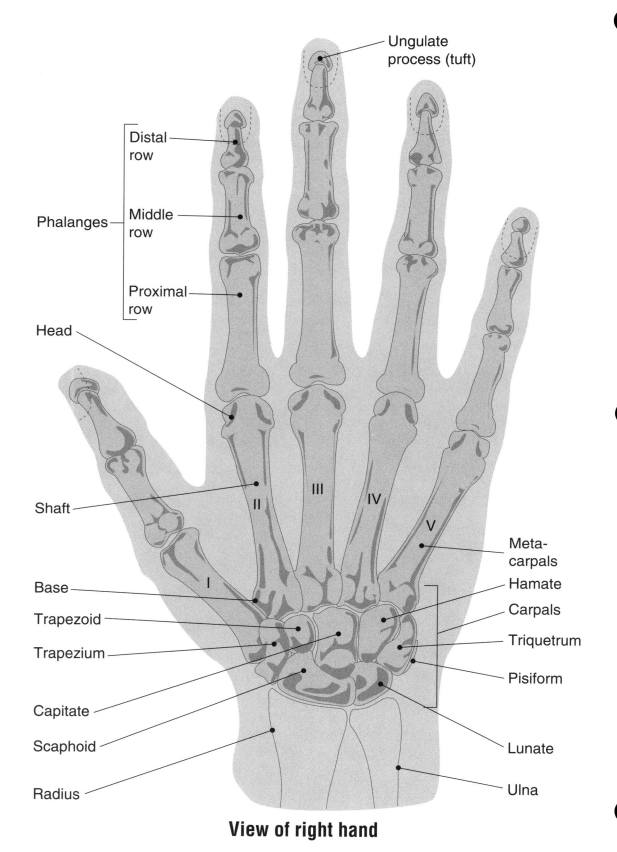

Ungulate
process (tuft)

Distal
row

Middle
row

Phalanges

Proximal
row

Head

Shaft

Base

Trapezoid

Trapezium

Capitate

Scaphoid

Radius

I

II

III

IV

V

Meta-
carpals

Hamate

Carpals

Triquetrum

Pisiform

Lunate

Ulna

View of right hand

Figure 5–3.

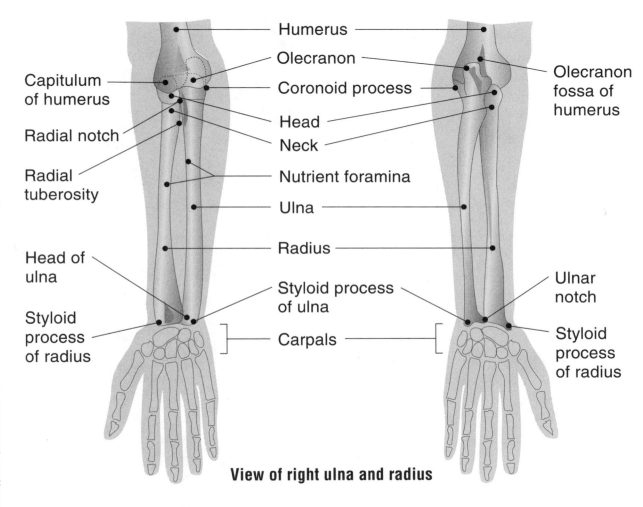

Capitulum of humerus

Radial notch

Radial tuberosity

Head of ulna

Styloid process of radius

Humerus

Olecranon

Coronoid process

Head

Neck

Nutrient foramina

Ulna

Radius

Styloid process of ulna

Carpals

Olecranon fossa of humerus

Ulnar notch

Styloid process of radius

View of right ulna and radius

Figure 5–6.

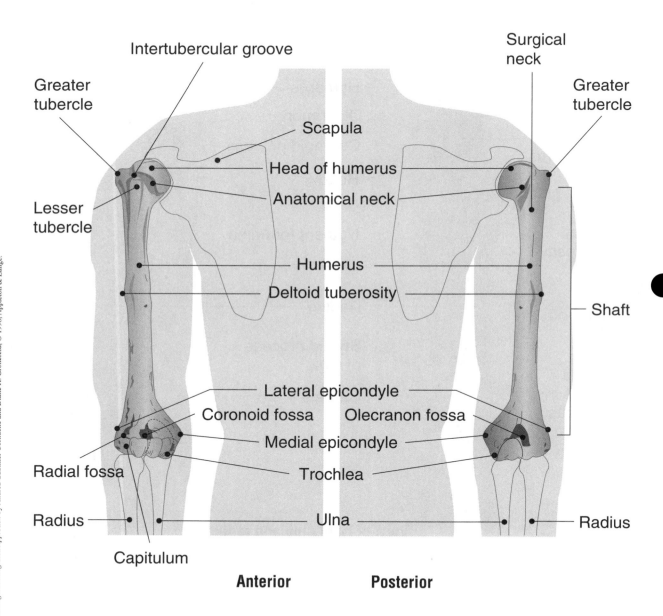

Greater
tubercle

Intertubercular groove

Surgical
neck

Greater
tubercle

Scapula

Head of humerus

Anatomical neck

Lesser
tubercle

Humerus

Deltoid tuberosity

Shaft

Lateral epicondyle

Coronoid fossa   Olecranon fossa

Medial epicondyle

Radial fossa

Trochlea

Radius   Ulna   Radius

Capitulum

Anterior   **Posterior**

Figure 5–7.

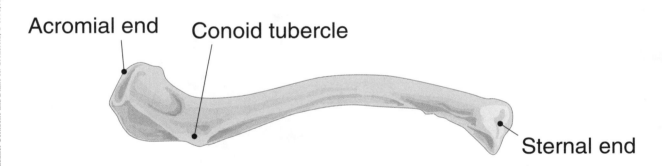

Acromial (lateral) end

Sternal (medial) end

Anterior

Acromial end

Conoid tubercle

Sternal end

Posterior

Figure 6–3.

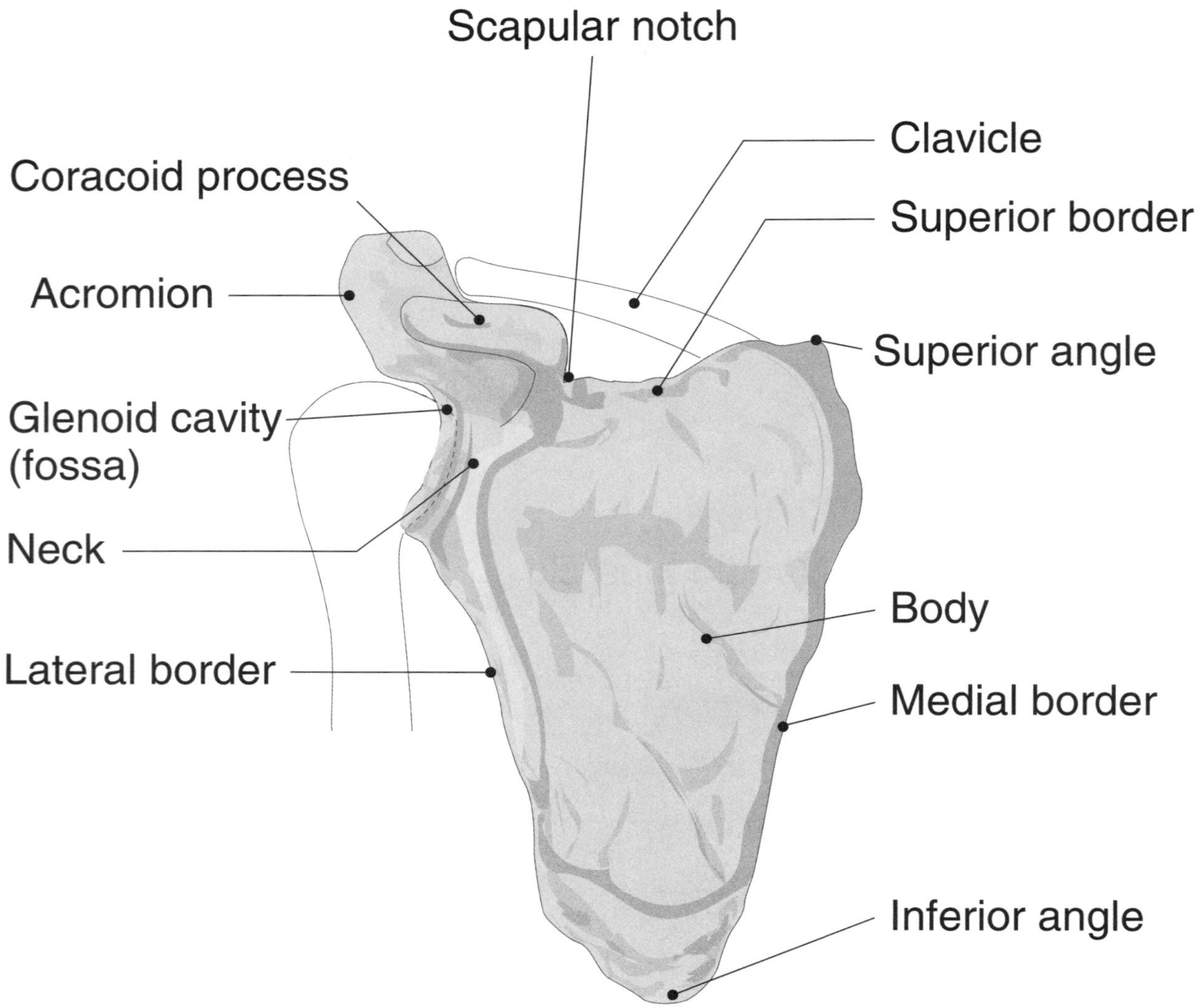

Scapular notch

Clavicle

Coracoid process

Superior border

Acromion

Superior angle

Glenoid cavity
(fossa)

Neck

Body

Lateral border

Medial border

Inferior angle

Figure 6–7A.

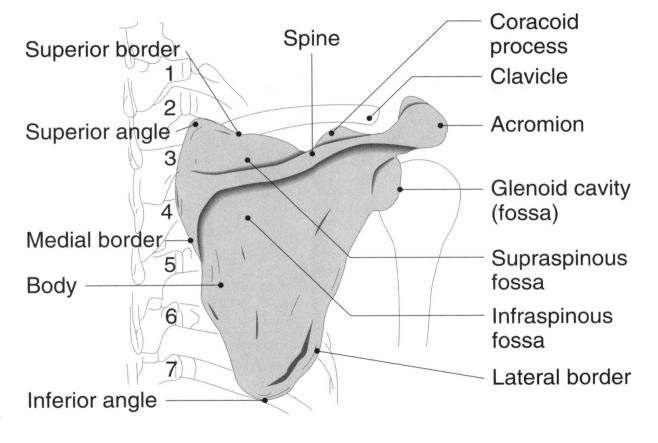

Superior border

Spine

Coracoid process

Clavicle

1

Superior angle

2

Acromion

3

Glenoid cavity (fossa)

4

Medial border

Supraspinous fossa

5

Body

Infraspinous fossa

6

7

Lateral border

Inferior angle

Figure 6–7B.

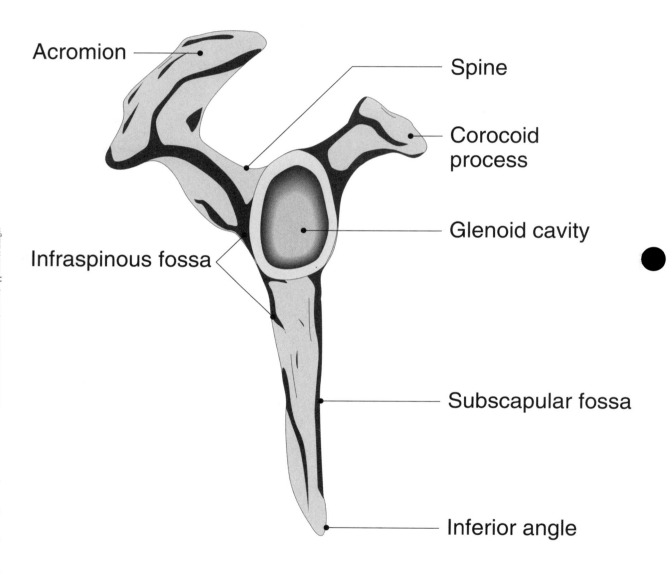

Acromion

Spine

Corocoid process

Glenoid cavity

Infraspinous fossa

Subscapular fossa

Inferior angle

Figure 6–7C.

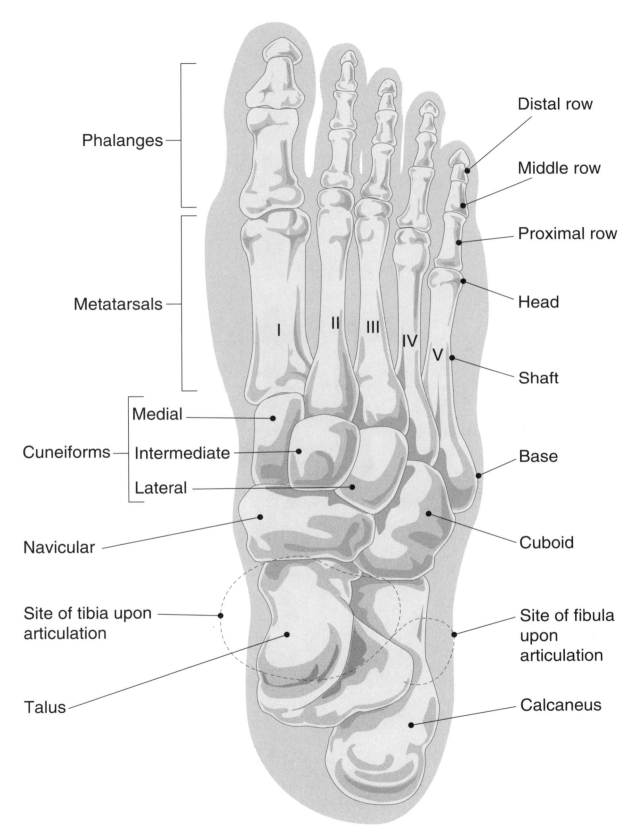

Phalanges

Metatarsals

Cuneiforms — Medial

Intermediate

Lateral

Navicular

Site of tibia upon articulation

Talus

Distal row

Middle row

Proximal row

Head

Shaft

Base

Cuboid

Site of fibula upon articulation

Calcaneus

I II III IV V

Figure 7–4.

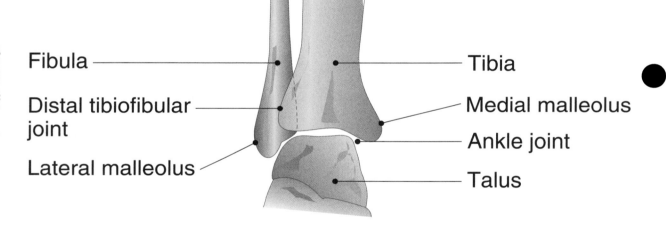

Fibula

Distal tibiofibular
joint

Lateral malleolus

Tibia

Medial malleolus

Ankle joint

Talus

Figure 7–5.

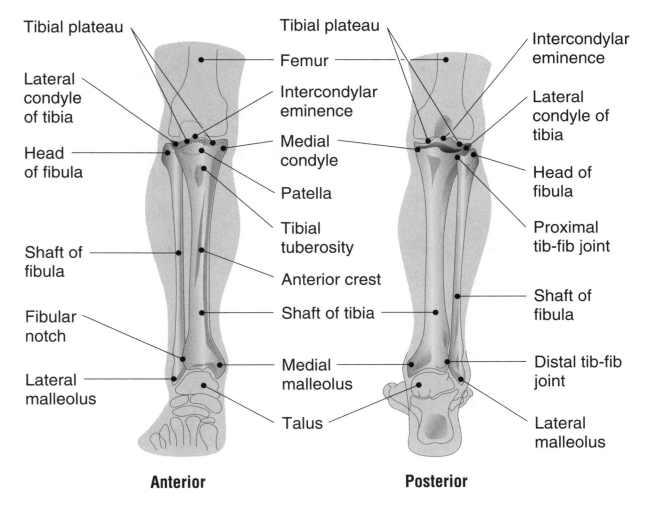

Tibial plateau

Lateral condyle of tibia

Head of fibula

Shaft of fibula

Fibular notch

Lateral malleolus

Tibial plateau

Femur

Intercondylar eminence

Medial condyle

Patella

Tibial tuberosity

Anterior crest

Shaft of tibia

Medial malleolus

Talus

Anterior

Tibial plateau

Intercondylar eminence

Lateral condyle of tibia

Head of fibula

Proximal tib-fib joint

Shaft of fibula

Distal tib-fib joint

Lateral malleolus

Posterior

Figure 7–8.

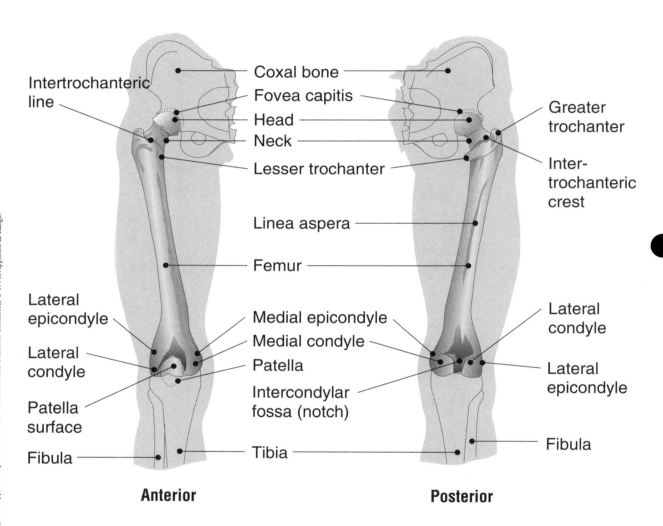

Intertrochanteric line

Coxal bone

Fovea capitis

Head

Neck

Lesser trochanter

Greater trochanter

Inter- trochanteric crest

Linea aspera

Femur

Lateral epicondyle

Lateral condyle

Patella surface

Fibula

Medial epicondyle

Medial condyle

Patella

Intercondylar fossa (notch)

Tibia

Lateral condyle

Lateral epicondyle

Fibula

Anterior

Posterior

Figure 7–10.

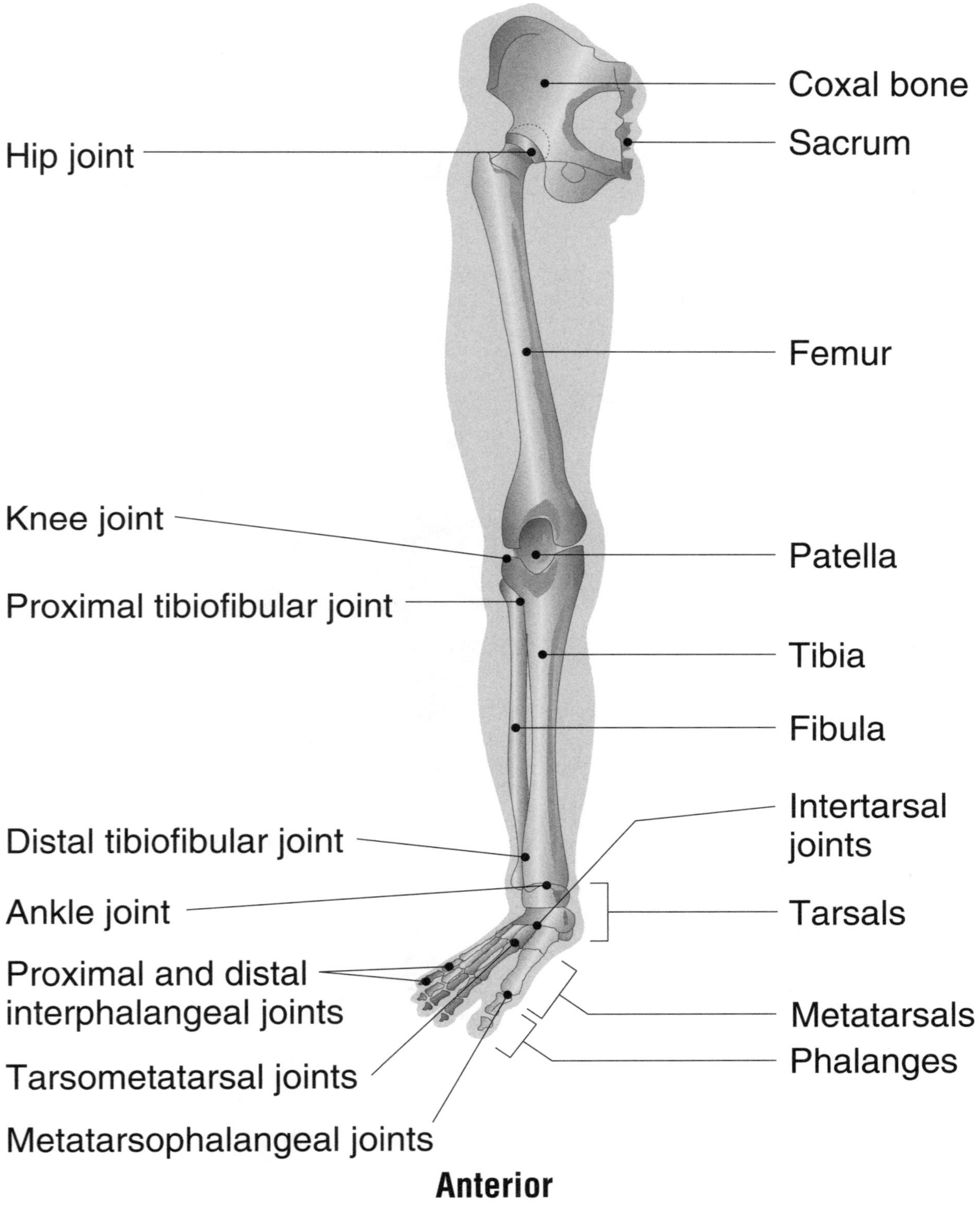

Coxal bone

Sacrum

Hip joint

Femur

Knee joint

Patella

Proximal tibiofibular joint

Tibia

Fibula

Intertarsal joints

Distal tibiofibular joint

Ankle joint

Tarsals

Proximal and distal interphalangeal joints

Metatarsals

Tarsometatarsal joints

Phalanges

Metatarsophalangeal joints

Anterior

Figure 7–15.

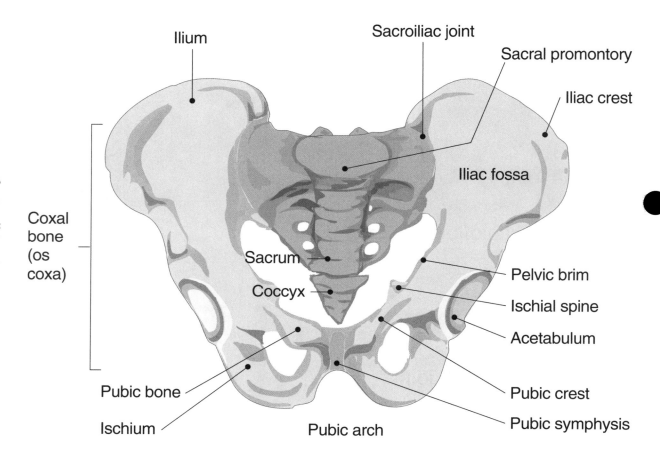

Ilium

Sacroiliac joint

Sacral promontory

Iliac crest

Iliac fossa

Coxal bone (os coxa)

Sacrum

Coccyx

Pelvic brim

Ischial spine

Acetabulum

Pubic bone

Ischium

Pubic crest

Pubic symphysis

Pubic arch

Figure 8–4A.

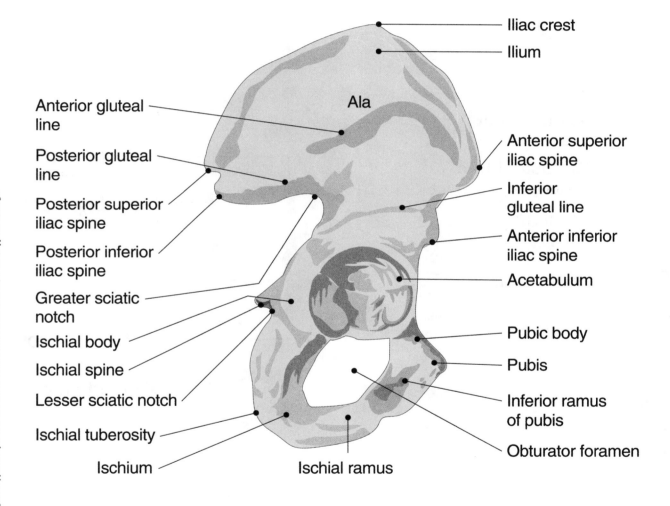

Iliac crest

Ilium

Ala

Anterior gluteal line

Posterior gluteal line

Posterior superior iliac spine

Posterior inferior iliac spine

Greater sciatic notch

Ischial body

Ischial spine

Lesser sciatic notch

Ischial tuberosity

Ischium

Ischial ramus

Anterior superior iliac spine

Inferior gluteal line

Anterior inferior iliac spine

Acetabulum

Pubic body

Pubis

Inferior ramus of pubis

Obturator foramen

Figure 8–4B.

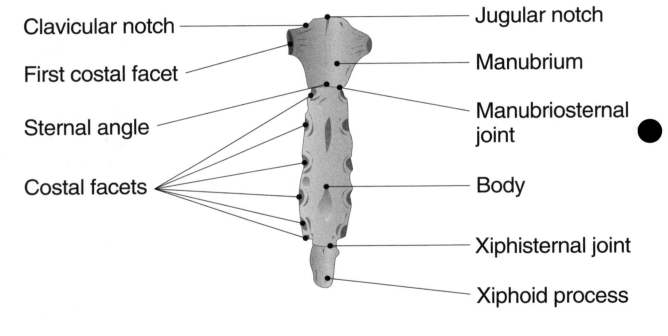

Clavicular notch

First costal facet

Sternal angle

Costal facets

Jugular notch

Manubrium

Manubriosternal
joint

Body

Xiphisternal joint

Xiphoid process

Figure 9–3.

Anterior

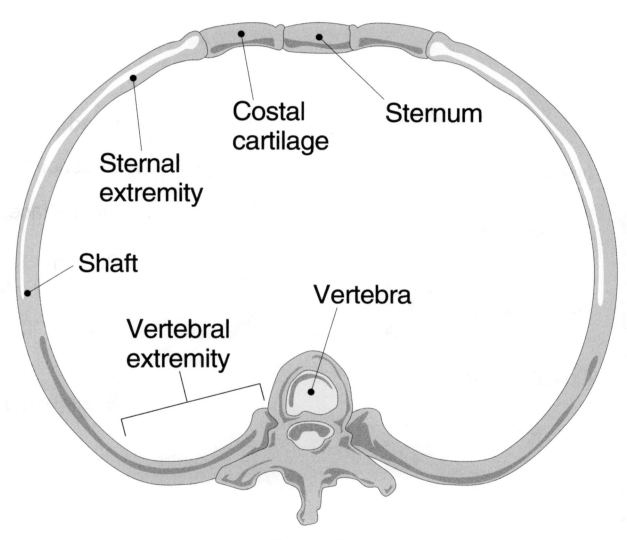

Costal
cartilage

Sternum

Sternal
extremity

Shaft

Vertebra

Vertebral
extremity

Posterior

Figure 9–4.

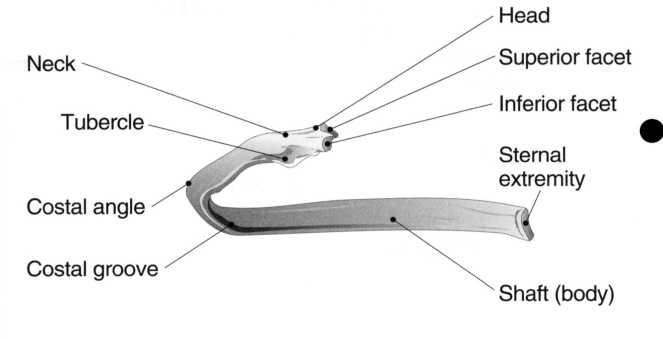

Neck

Tubercle

Costal angle

Costal groove

Head

Superior facet

Inferior facet

Sternal extremity

Shaft (body)

Figure 9–5.

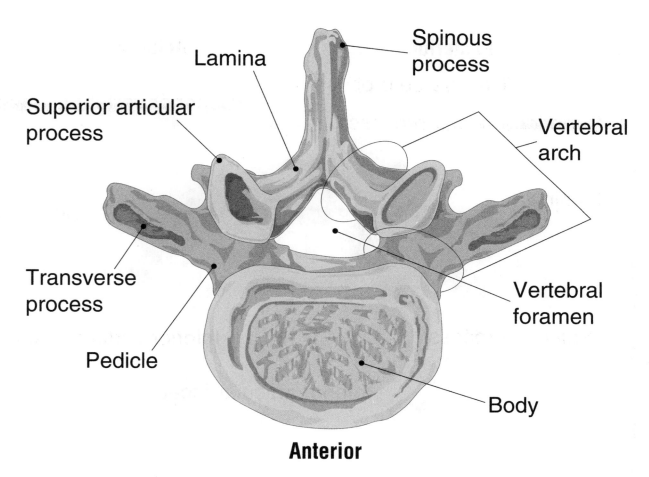

Posterior

Spinous process

Lamina

Superior articular process

Vertebral arch

Transverse process

Vertebral foramen

Pedicle

Body

Anterior

Figure 10–5A.

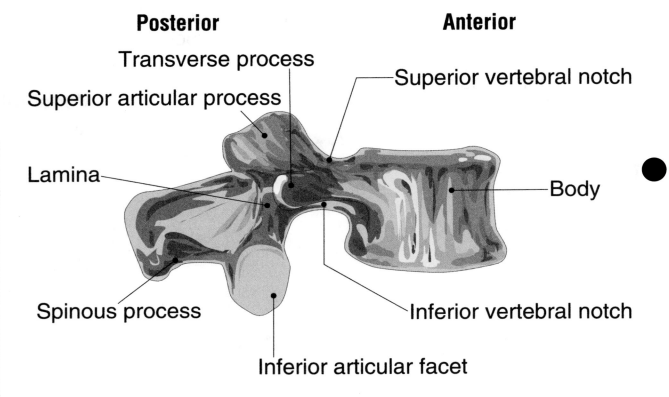

Posterior **Anterior**

Transverse process

Superior articular process

Superior vertebral notch

Lamina

Body

Spinous process

Inferior vertebral notch

Inferior articular facet

Figure 10–5B.

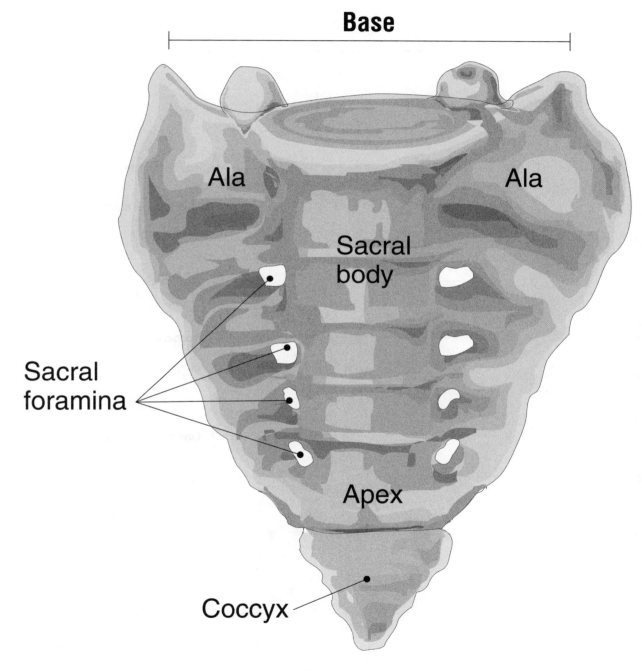

Base

Ala

Ala

Sacral body

Sacral foramina

Apex

Coccyx

Figure 10–12.

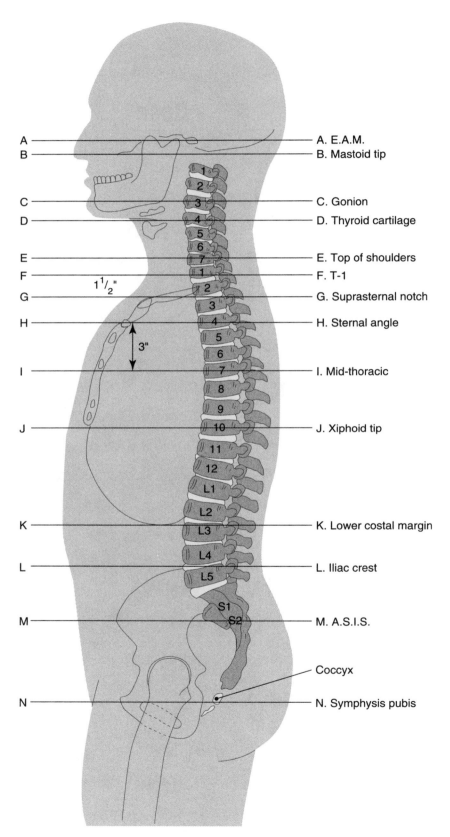

A — A. E.A.M.
B — B. Mastoid tip

C — C. Gonion
D — D. Thyroid cartilage

E — E. Top of shoulders
F — F. T-1
G — G. Suprasternal notch
H — H. Sternal angle

I — I. Mid-thoracic

J — J. Xiphoid tip

K — K. Lower costal margin

L — L. Iliac crest

M — M. A.S.I.S.

Coccyx

N — N. Symphysis pubis

$1\frac{1}{2}$"

3"

Figure 10–21.

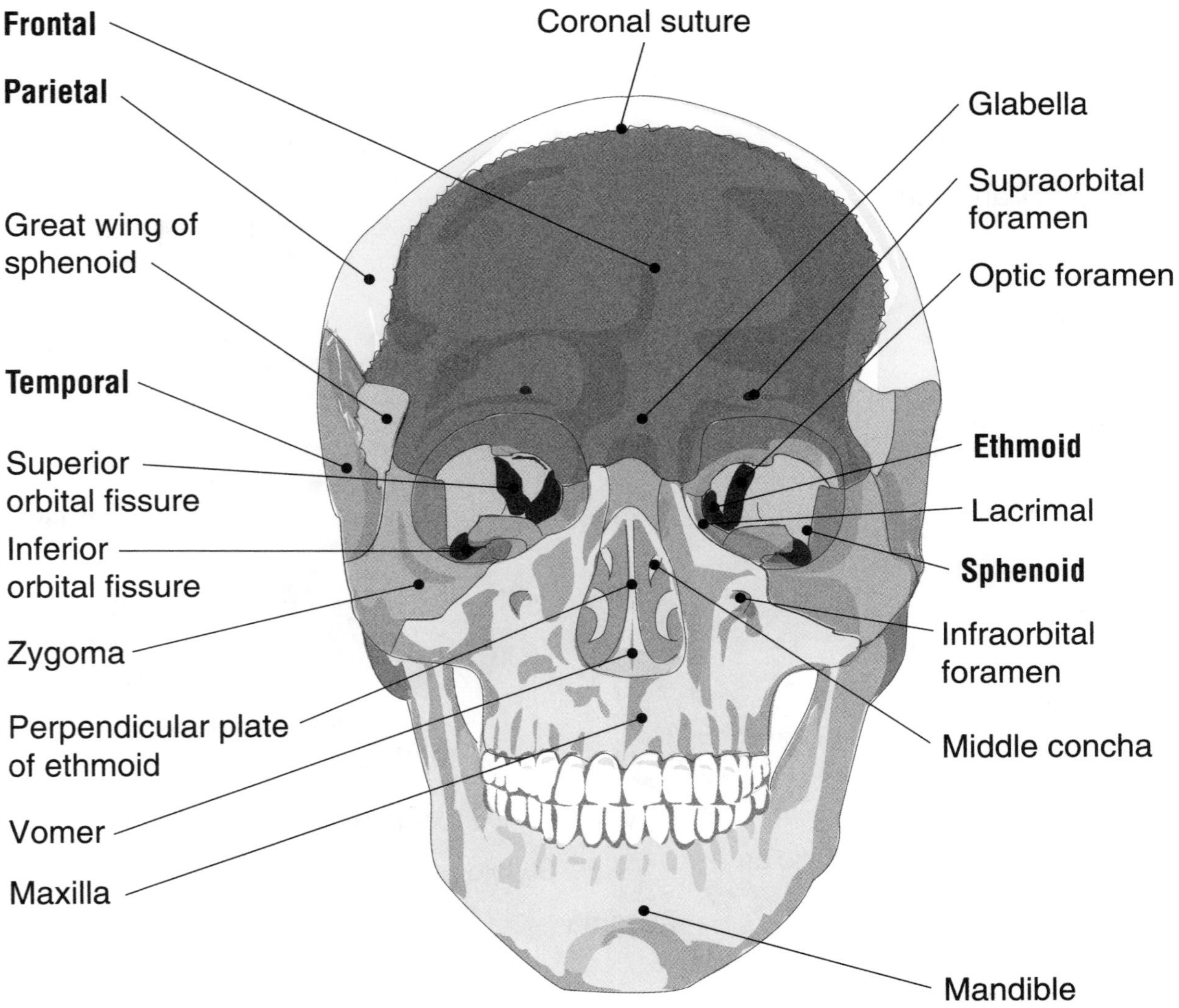

Frontal

Parietal

Great wing of
sphenoid

Temporal

Superior
orbital fissure

Inferior
orbital fissure

Zygoma

Perpendicular plate
of ethmoid

Vomer

Maxilla

Coronal suture

Glabella

Supraorbital
foramen

Optic foramen

Ethmoid

Lacrimal

Sphenoid

Infraorbital
foramen

Middle concha

Mandible

Figure 11–2A.

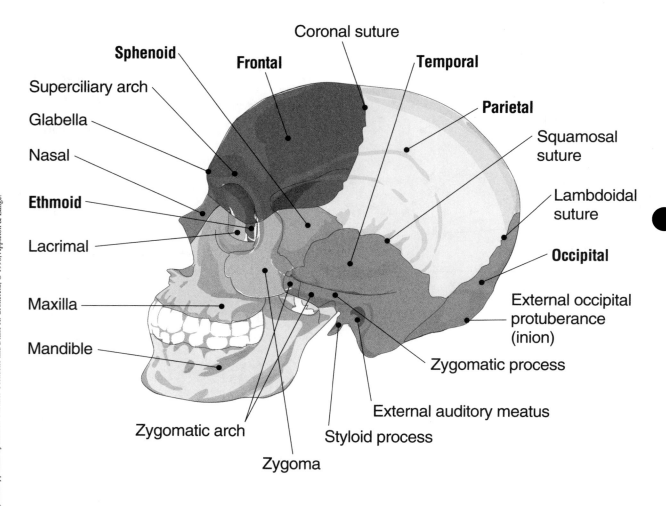

Coronal suture

Sphenoid

Frontal

Temporal

Superciliary arch

Parietal

Glabella

Squamosal
suture

Nasal

Lambdoidal
suture

Ethmoid

Occipital

Lacrimal

External occipital
protuberance
(inion)

Maxilla

Mandible

Zygomatic process

External auditory meatus

Zygomatic arch

Styloid process

Zygoma

Figure 11–2B.

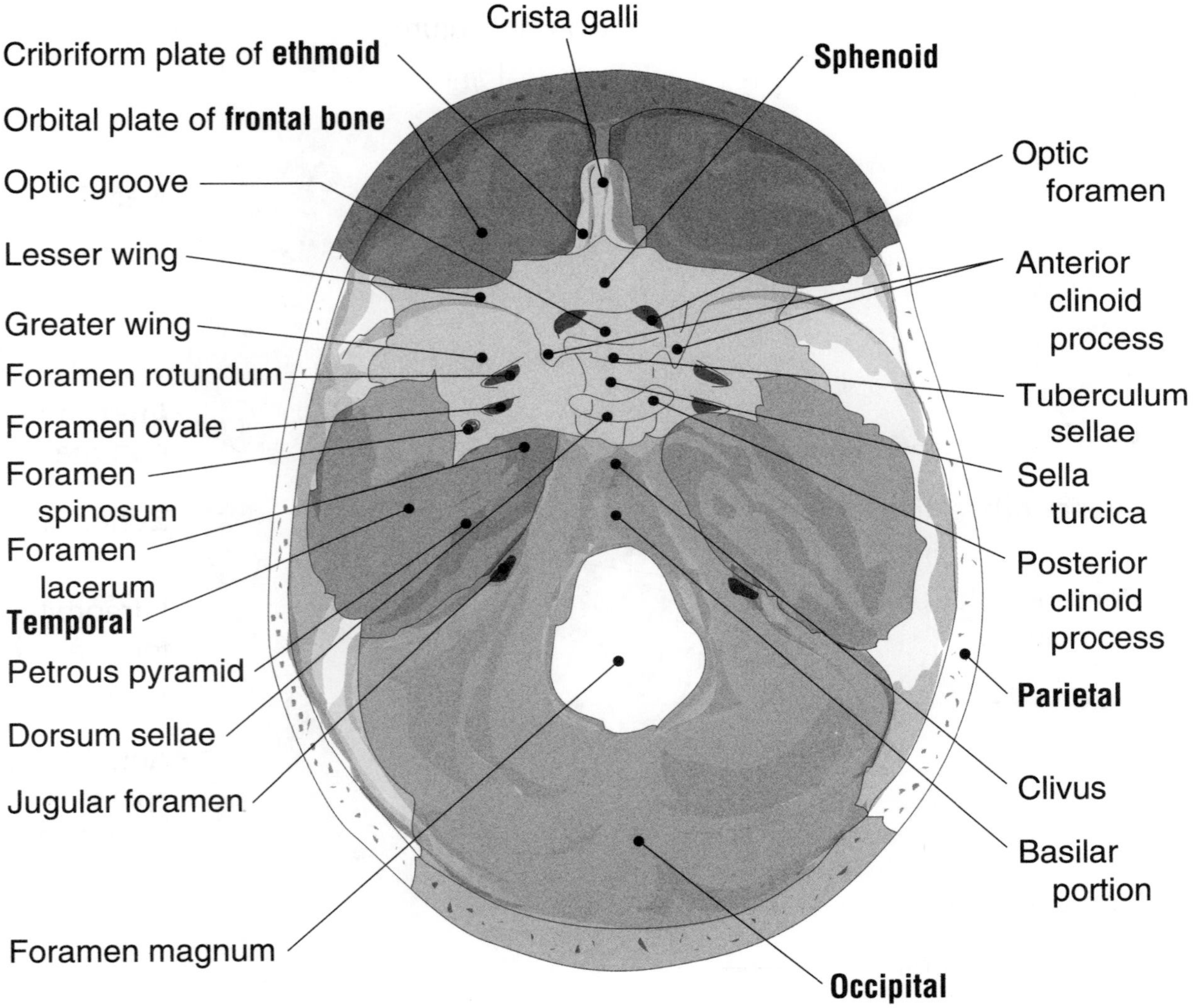

Crista galli

Cribriform plate of **ethmoid**

Orbital plate of **frontal bone**

Optic groove

Lesser wing

Greater wing

Foramen rotundum

Foramen ovale

Foramen spinosum

Foramen lacerum

Temporal

Petrous pyramid

Dorsum sellae

Jugular foramen

Foramen magnum

Sphenoid

Optic foramen

Anterior clinoid process

Tuberculum sellae

Sella turcica

Posterior clinoid process

Parietal

Clivus

Basilar portion

Occipital

Figure 11–2C.

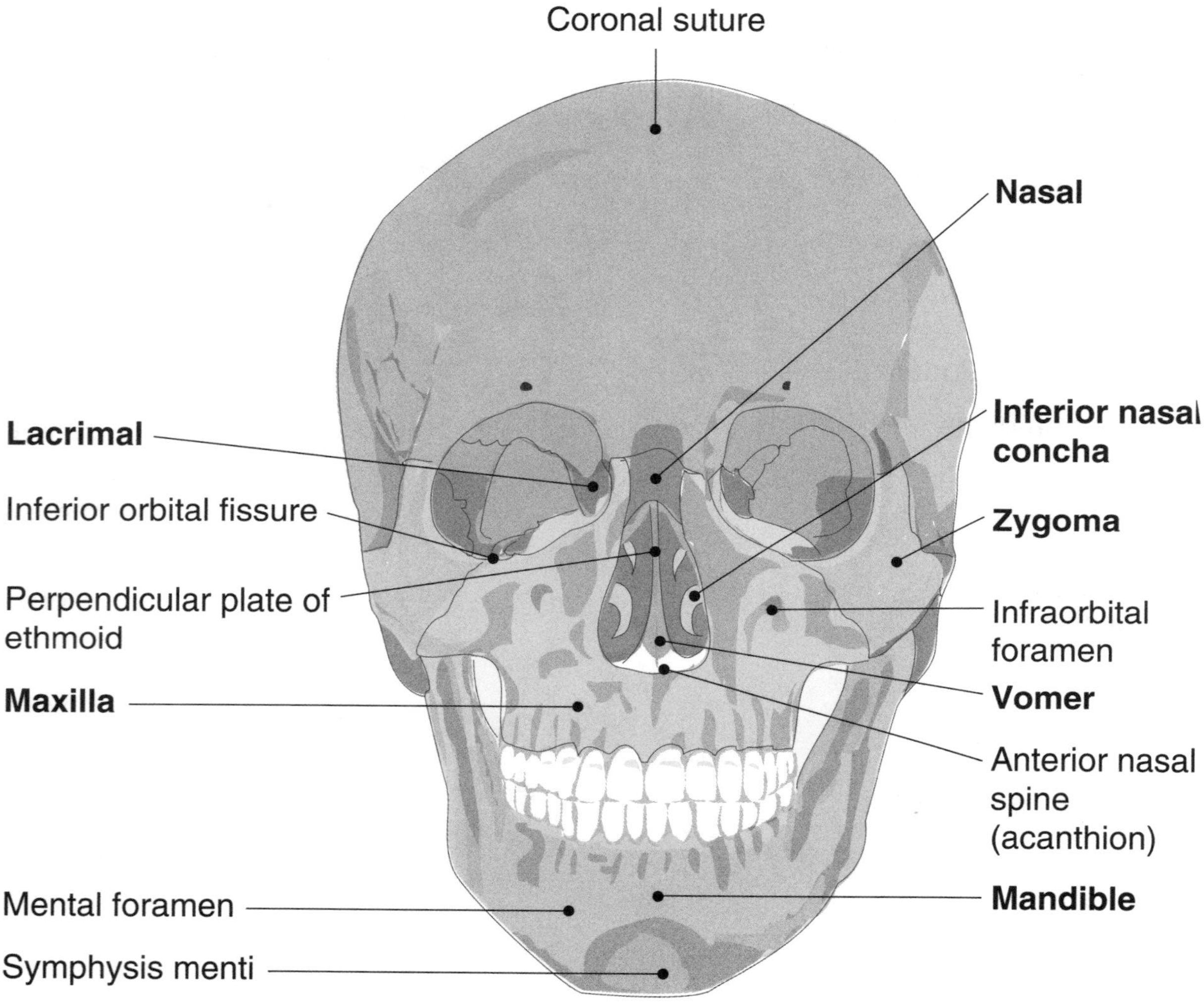

Coronal suture

Nasal

Inferior nasal concha

Zygoma

Infraorbital foramen

Vomer

Anterior nasal spine (acanthion)

Mandible

Lacrimal

Inferior orbital fissure

Perpendicular plate of ethmoid

Maxilla

Mental foramen

Symphysis menti

Figure 12–2A.

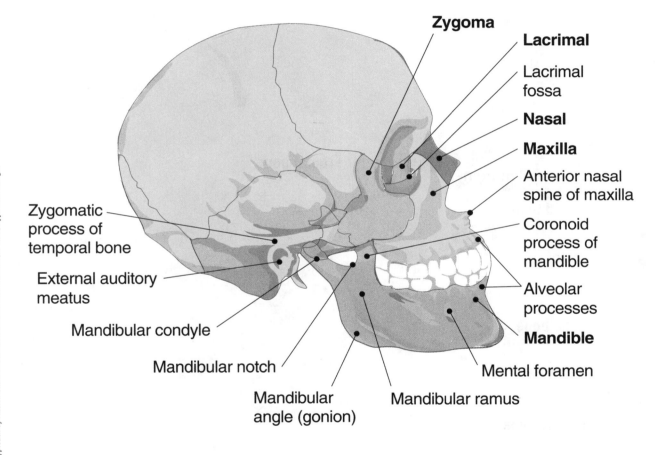

Zygoma

Lacrimal

Lacrimal
fossa

Nasal

Maxilla

Anterior nasal
spine of maxilla

Coronoid
process of
mandible

Alveolar
processes

Mandible

Mental foramen

Mandibular ramus

Mandibular
angle (gonion)

Mandibular notch

Mandibular condyle

External auditory
meatus

Zygomatic
process of
temporal bone

Figure 12–2B.

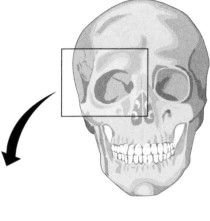

Frontal bone

Supraorbital margin

Sphenoid bone

Superior orbital
fissure

Palatine bone

Inferior orbital
fissure

Zygomatic bone

Infraorbital foramen

Supraorbital
foramen

Optic foramen

Nasal bone

Lacrimal bone

Ethmoid bone

Maxilla

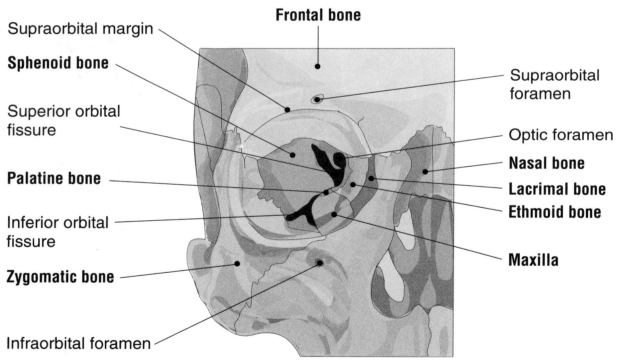

Figure 12–15.

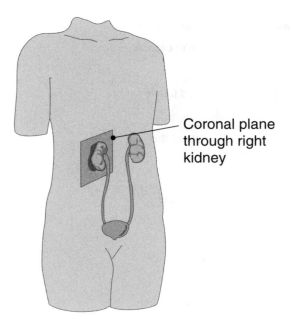

Coronal plane through right kidney

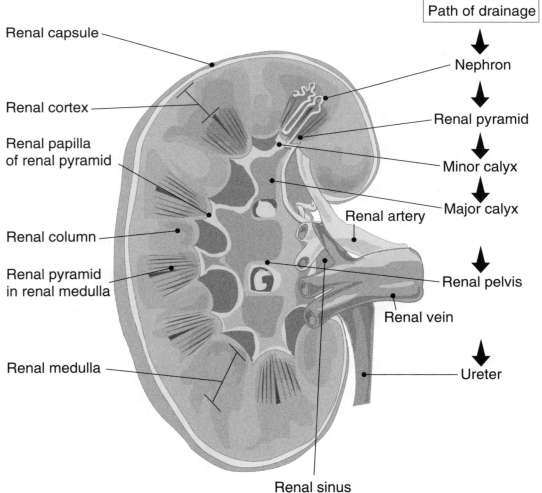

Path of drainage

Nephron

Renal pyramid

Minor calyx

Major calyx

Renal pelvis

Ureter

Renal capsule

Renal cortex

Renal papilla of renal pyramid

Renal column

Renal pyramid in renal medulla

Renal medulla

Renal artery

Renal vein

Renal sinus

Figure 14–4.

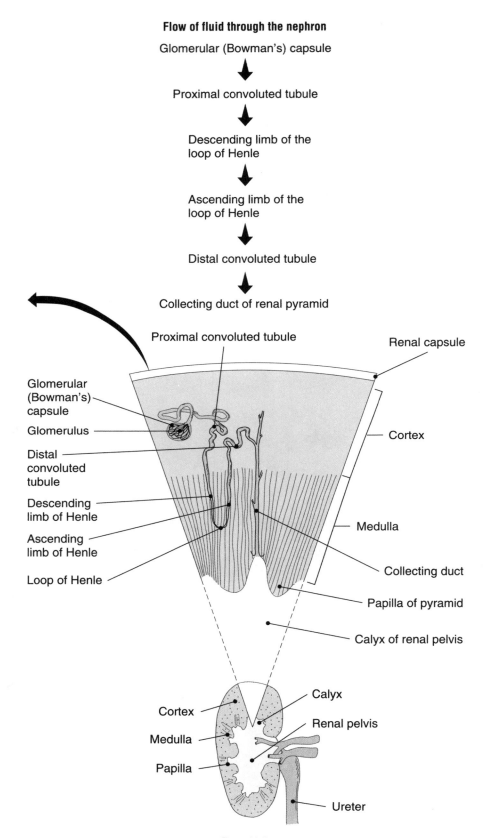

Flow of fluid through the nephron

Glomerular (Bowman's) capsule

↓

Proximal convoluted tubule

↓

Descending limb of the loop of Henle

↓

Ascending limb of the loop of Henle

↓

Distal convoluted tubule

↓

Collecting duct of renal pyramid

Proximal convoluted tubule

Renal capsule

Glomerular (Bowman's) capsule

Glomerulus

Cortex

Distal convoluted tubule

Descending limb of Henle

Ascending limb of Henle

Medulla

Loop of Henle

Collecting duct

Papilla of pyramid

Calyx of renal pelvis

Cortex

Calyx

Medulla

Renal pelvis

Papilla

Ureter

Figure 14–6.

From *Radiographic Anatomy & Positioning: An Integrated Approach* by Andrea Gauthier Cornuelle and Diane H. Gronefeld, © 1998, Appleton & Lange.

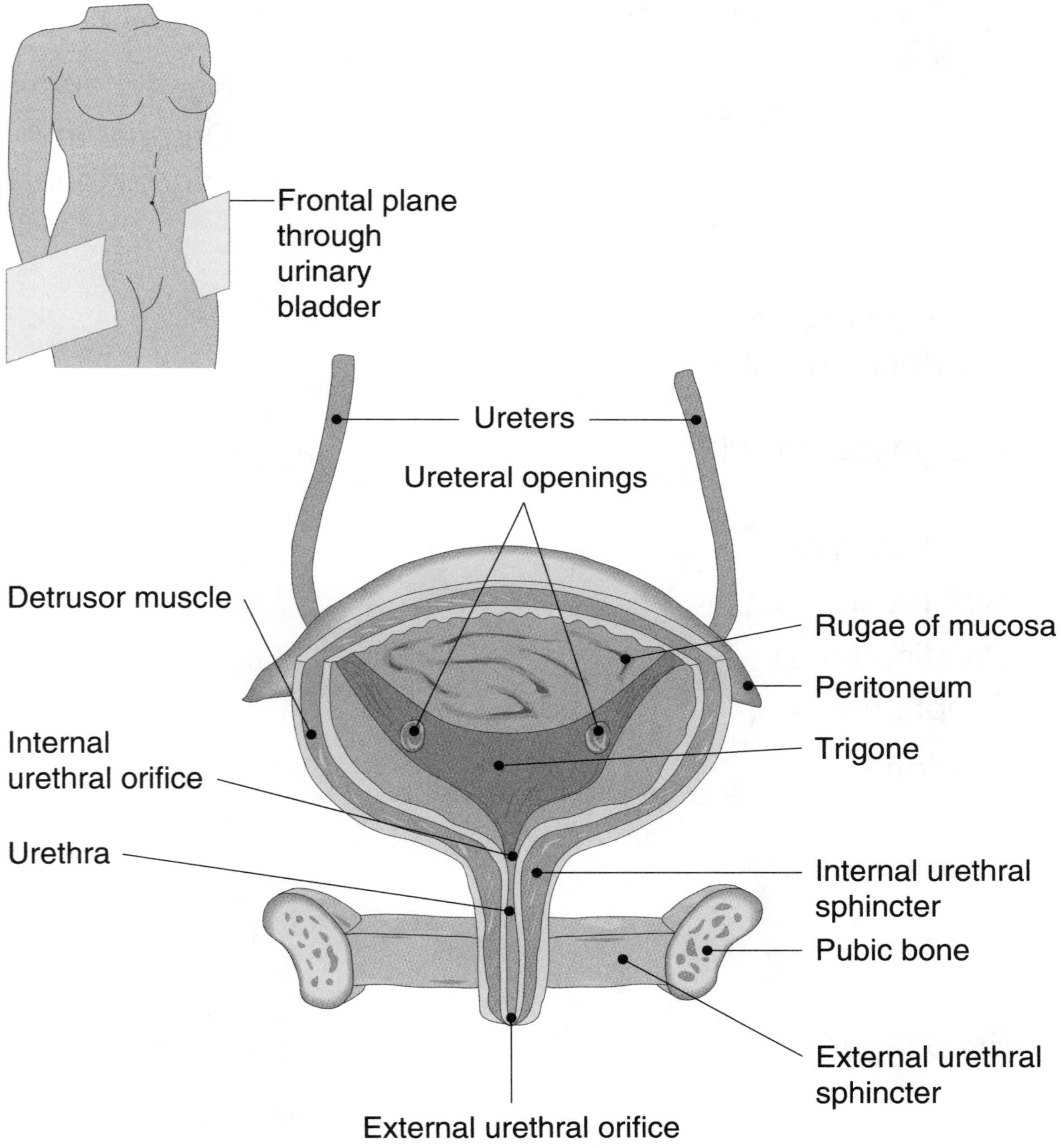

Frontal plane through urinary bladder

Ureters

Ureteral openings

Detrusor muscle

Rugae of mucosa

Peritoneum

Internal urethral orifice

Trigone

Urethra

Internal urethral sphincter

Pubic bone

External urethral sphincter

External urethral orifice

Figure 14–11.

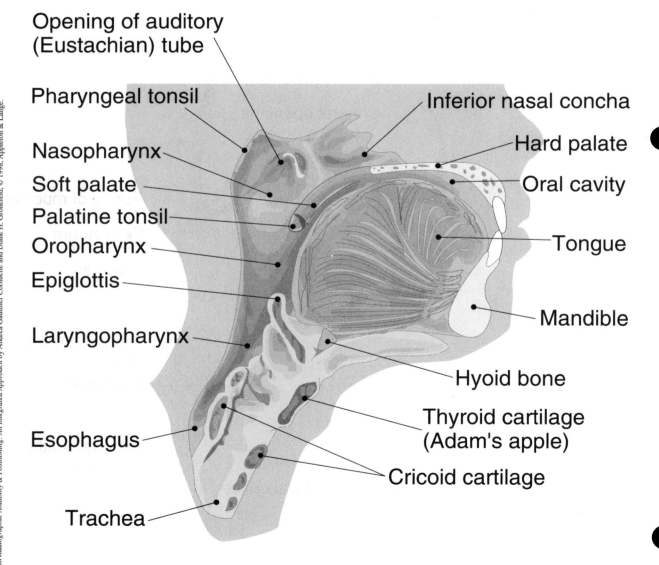

Superior

Sagittal plane through head and neck

Anterior

☐ Nasopharynx
■ Oropharynx
☐ Laryngopharynx

Opening of auditory (Eustachian) tube

Pharyngeal tonsil

Inferior nasal concha

Nasopharynx

Hard palate

Soft palate

Oral cavity

Palatine tonsil

Oropharynx

Tongue

Epiglottis

Laryngopharynx

Mandible

Hyoid bone

Thyroid cartilage (Adam's apple)

Esophagus

Cricoid cartilage

Trachea

Figure 15–7.

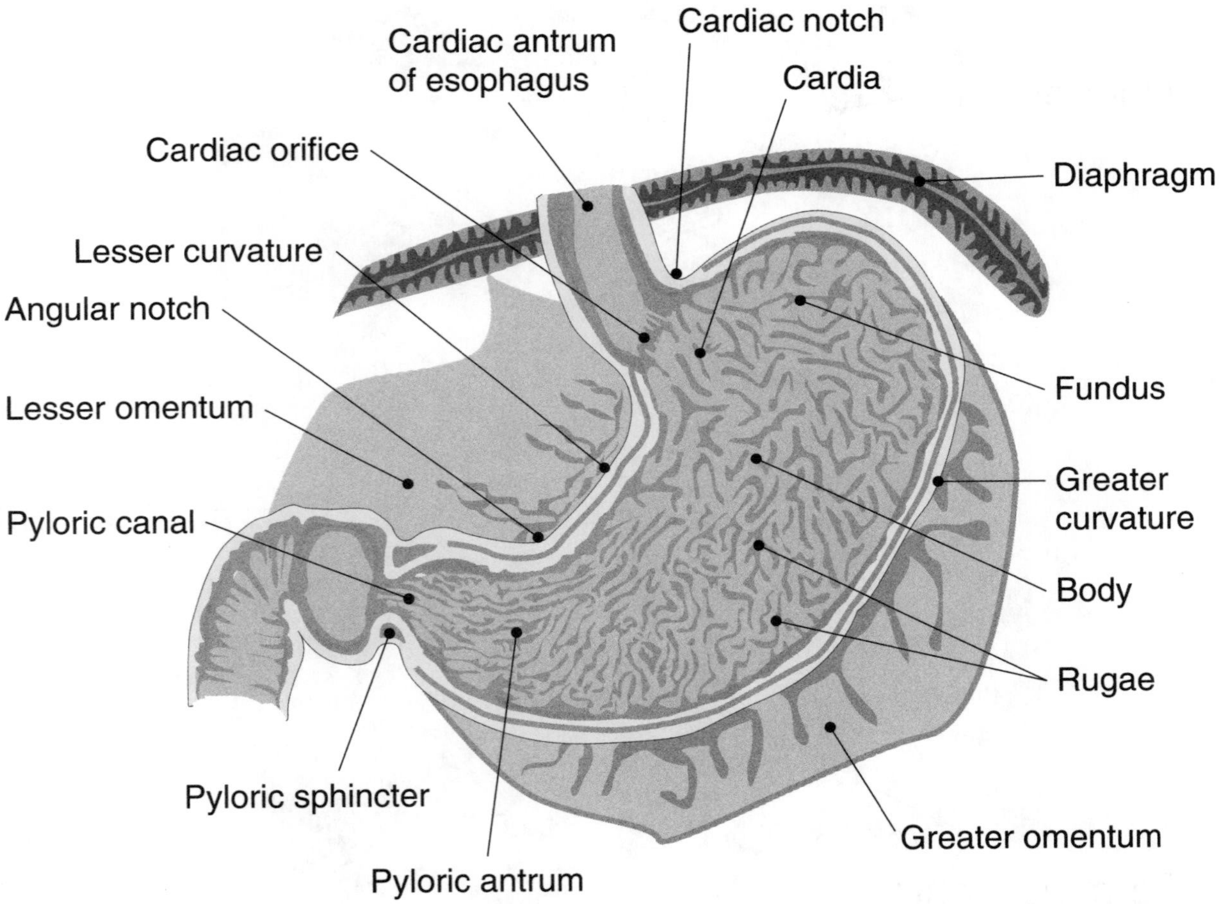

Cardiac antrum
of esophagus

Cardiac notch

Cardiac orifice

Cardia

Diaphragm

Lesser curvature

Angular notch

Fundus

Lesser omentum

Greater
curvature

Pyloric canal

Body

Rugae

Pyloric sphincter

Greater omentum

Pyloric antrum

Figure 15–11.

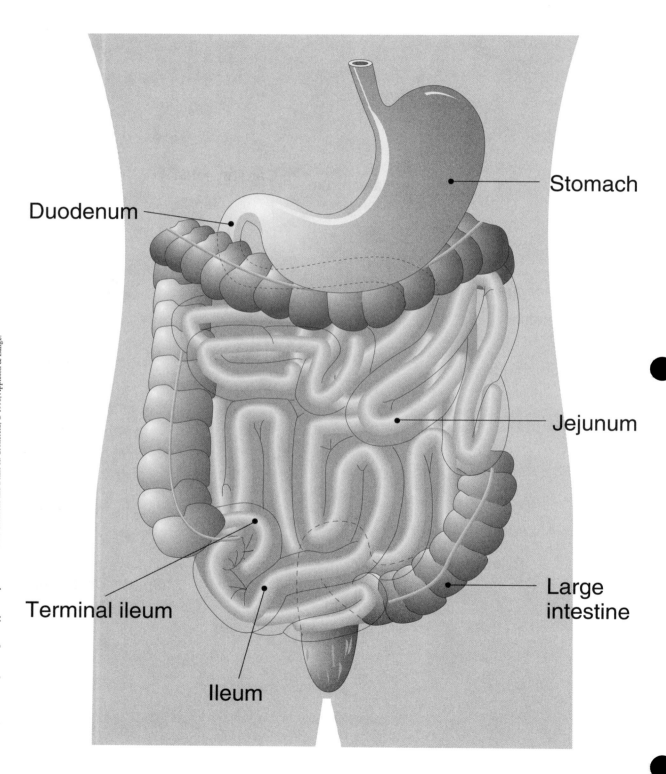

Stomach

Duodenum

Jejunum

Terminal ileum

Large
intestine

Ileum

Figure 15–14.

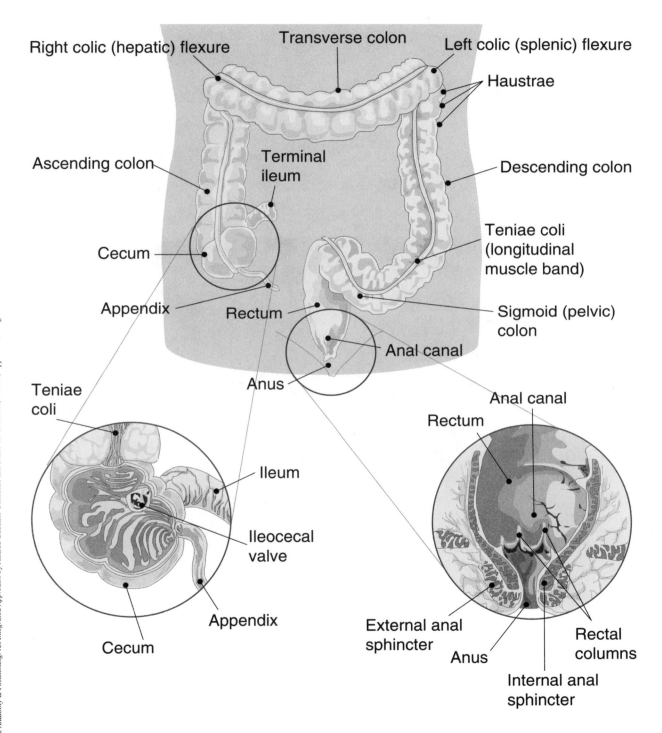

Right colic (hepatic) flexure

Transverse colon

Left colic (splenic) flexure

Haustrae

Ascending colon

Terminal ileum

Descending colon

Cecum

Teniae coli (longitudinal muscle band)

Appendix

Rectum

Sigmoid (pelvic) colon

Anal canal

Anus

Teniae coli

Anal canal

Rectum

Ileum

Ileocecal valve

Appendix

Cecum

External anal sphincter

Anus

Rectal columns

Internal anal sphincter

Figure 15–19.

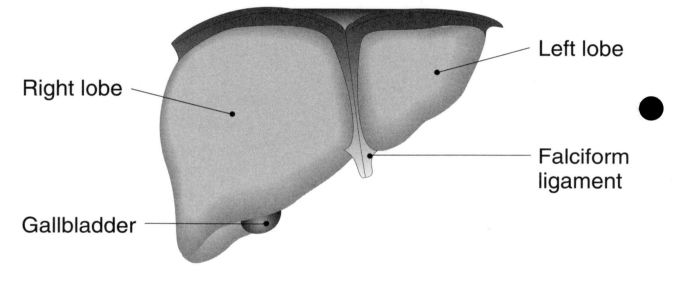

Right lobe

Left lobe

Falciform
ligament

Gallbladder

Figure 16–2.

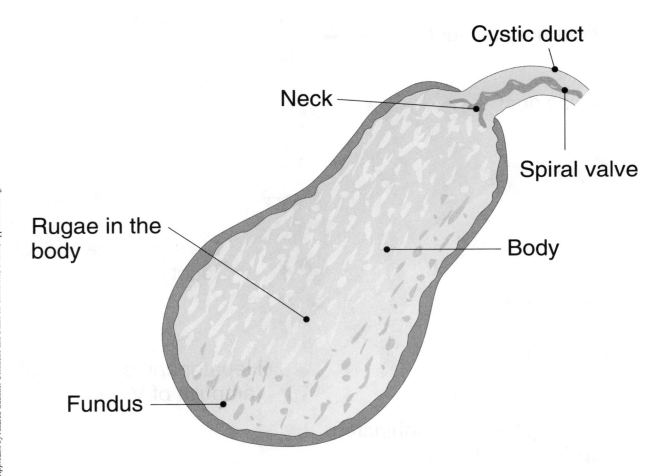

Cystic duct

Neck

Spiral valve

Rugae in the
body

Body

Fundus

Figure 16–8.

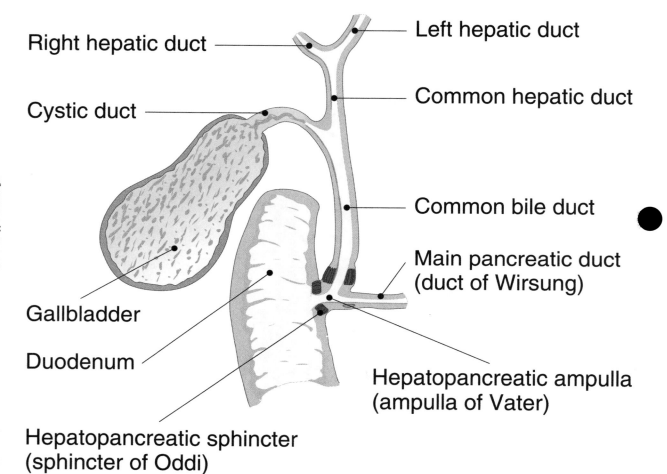

Right hepatic duct

Left hepatic duct

Cystic duct

Common hepatic duct

Common bile duct

Main pancreatic duct
(duct of Wirsung)

Gallbladder

Duodenum

Hepatopancreatic ampulla
(ampulla of Vater)

Hepatopancreatic sphincter
(sphincter of Oddi)

Figure 16–10.

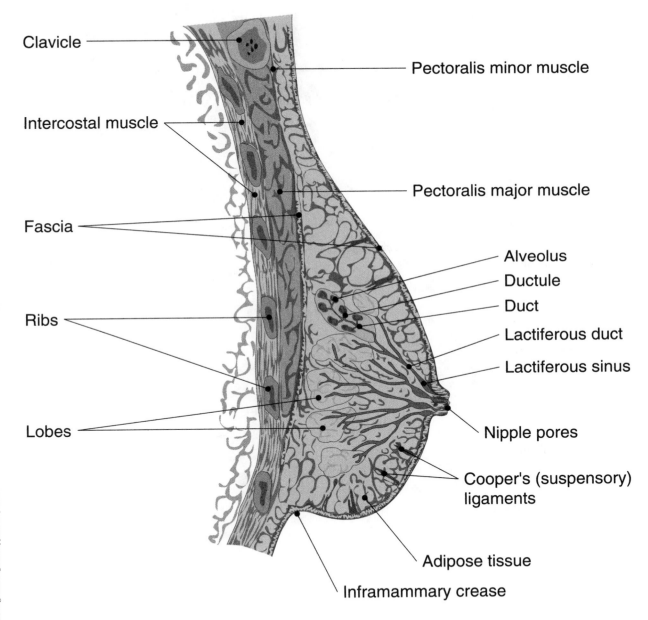

Clavicle

Intercostal muscle

Fascia

Ribs

Lobes

Pectoralis minor muscle

Pectoralis major muscle

Alveolus
Ductule
Duct
Lactiferous duct
Lactiferous sinus

Nipple pores

Cooper's (suspensory) ligaments

Adipose tissue
Inframammary crease

Figure 17–3.

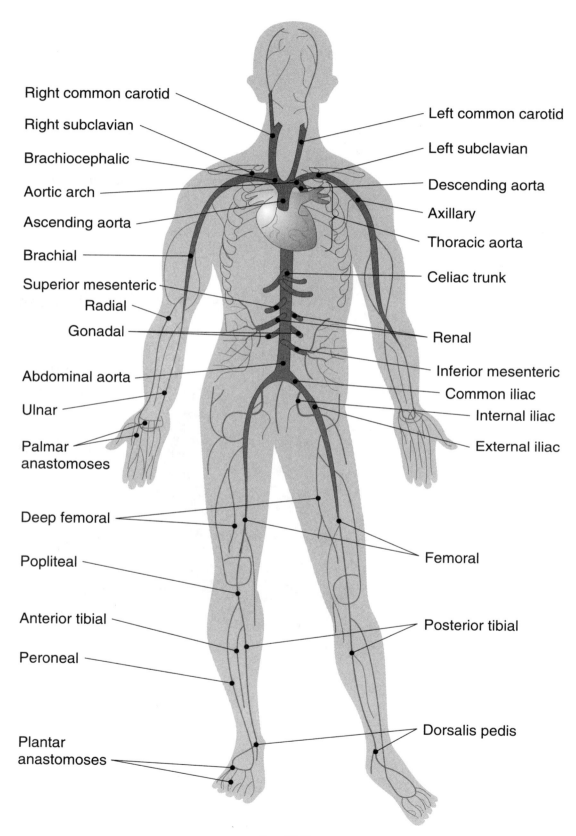

Right common carotid

Right subclavian

Brachiocephalic

Aortic arch

Ascending aorta

Brachial

Superior mesenteric

Radial

Gonadal

Abdominal aorta

Ulnar

Palmar
anastomoses

Deep femoral

Popliteal

Anterior tibial

Peroneal

Plantar
anastomoses

Left common carotid

Left subclavian

Descending aorta

Axillary

Thoracic aorta

Celiac trunk

Renal

Inferior mesenteric

Common iliac

Internal iliac

External iliac

Femoral

Posterior tibial

Dorsalis pedis

Figure 18–5A.

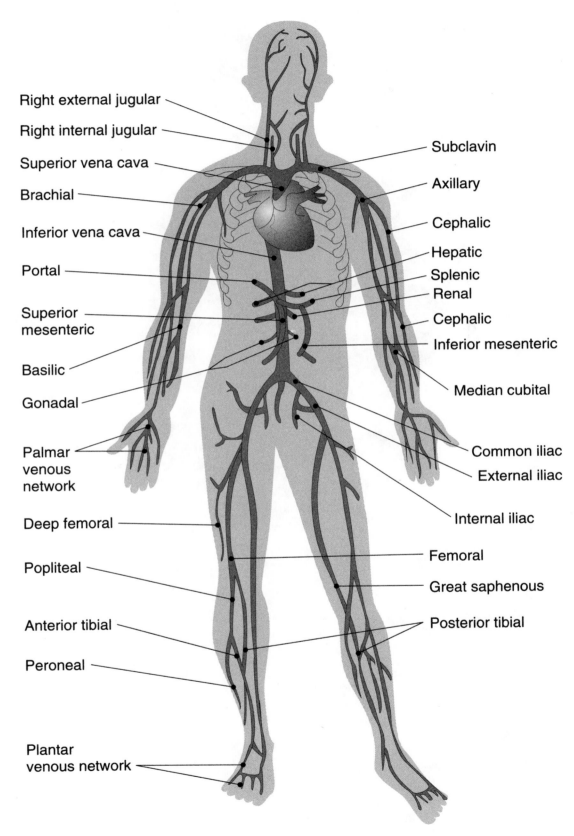

Right external jugular

Right internal jugular

Superior vena cava

Brachial

Inferior vena cava

Portal

Superior mesenteric

Basilic

Gonadal

Palmar venous network

Deep femoral

Popliteal

Anterior tibial

Peroneal

Plantar venous network

Subclavin

Axillary

Cephalic

Hepatic

Splenic

Renal

Cephalic

Inferior mesenteric

Median cubital

Common iliac

External iliac

Internal iliac

Femoral

Great saphenous

Posterior tibial

Figure 18–5B.